Vagus Nerve

and

Polyvagal Theory

Copyright © 2019

Table of Contents

Introduction

The nervous system is a part of an animal that is highly complex and is in charge of coordinating its actions and sensory information by transmitting information that travels as electrical impulses at a very high speed to and from different parts of its body. The nervous system is in charge of the detection of environmental changes that have an impact on the body, working hand in hand with the endocrine system to respond to such events.

In vertebrates, the nervous system is made up of two main parts, namely; the central nervous system (CNS) and the peripheral nervous system (PNS).

The Central Nervous System (CNS) consists of the brain and spinal cord while the Peripheral Nervous System (PNS) is made up mainly of nerves, which are enclosed bundles of the long thin fibers called axons, that connect the Central Nervous System to every other part of the body.

The cell is the simplest unit of life.Thus, we can say that everything is composed of this basic form.

The nervous system at the cellular level, in other words, in its basic form, is defined by the presence of a special type of cell, called the nerve cell also known as a "neuron"

Neurons are made up of special structures that permit them to send signals rapidly and precisely to other cells.

They send signals "precisely" because they are directly connected to the supposed cells while they send signals "rapidly" because they send them in the form of electrochemical waves which travel along their structurally thin fibers called axons which cause neurotransmitters to be released at junctions called synapses.

A cell may be excited, modulated or inhibited when it receives a synaptic signal from a neuron.

Neurons work together in transmitting information to and from the brain and they do that by connections that can form neural pathways, neural circuits, and larger networks to generate an organism's perception of the world and determine its reaction to it. Alongside neurons, the nervous system also contains other specialized cells called glial cells (or simply glia), which provide support, metabolically or structurally.

Nerves are also classified according to their functions. They are of two types;

1. Sensory or afferent are nerves that detect external contact and effects on the body and transmit signals from the body to the Central Nervous System (CNS)

2. Motor or efferent nerves are nerves that transmit information from the Central Nervous System (CNS) to targeted muscles or tissues.

In the peripheral nervous system. Nerves make the provision of a common pathway for the electrochemical nerve impulses (signals) called "action potentials" that are transmitted along each of the structurally long thin fibers known as "axon" to peripheral organs or, in the case of sensory nerves, from there back to the central nervous system (CNS). The nerve has specialized structures which include; The axon-which is an extension of a sole neuron-andother supportive cells such as Schwann cells-that coat the axons in myelin-, the dendrites, etc.

The Peripheral Nervous System is further divided into three distinct systems, namely; the somatic, autonomic, and enteric nervous systems. Somatic nerves balance voluntary movement. The autonomic nervous system is further divided into subsystems which are; the sympathetic and the parasympathetic nervous systems.the sympathetic nervous system, is stimulated in response to emergencies to mobilize energy, while the parasympathetic nervous system is stimulated when the organisms are in a relaxed state. The enteric nervous system is responsible for regulating the gastrointestinal system. The systems that function involuntarily are the autonomic and enteric nervous systems while the Somatic nervous system functions voluntarily.

Nerves are divided into two;

1. Cranial Nerves: These are Nerves that have its origin from the "cranium", terminating at different locations in the body thus the name; cranial nerves.

2. Spinal Nerves: They are called spinal nerves because they are nerves that originate from the spinal cord, terminating at different locations of the body. They are called mixed nerves because they serve both motor and sensory functions.

The cranial nerves;

are pairs of nerves that originate in the brain and terminate at different parts of the head, neck, and abdomen. There are 12 of them, each named in accordance with their function or structure.

According to their location from the front part of the brain to the back part of the brain, each nerve has a corresponding Roman numeral between I and XII. For example, the olfactory nerve is closest to the front of your head, so it's designated as "I" while the hypoglossal nerve is closest to the back part of the brain and the farthest to the front part of the brain and thus is designated as 'XII".

Their functions are mainly categorized as being either sensory or motor. The sensory nerves are involved with your senses, such as smell, sight, hearing, and touch while the motor nerves control the movement and function of muscles or glands.

The 12 cranial nerves

I. The olfactory nerve is responsible for the transmission of sensory information to your brain regarding smells that you encounter.

II. The optic nerve regulates human vision.

III. The oculomotor nerve has muscle function and pupil response, as its two distinct motor functions:

IV. The trochlear nerve works to supervise the superior oblique muscle that then controls the downward and upward movement of the eyes.

V. The trigeminal nerve is known as the largest of your cranial nerves with both sensory and motor functions.

VI. The abducens nerve controls another muscle called the "lateral rectus" muscle that is associated with eye movement,

VII. The facial nerve contains both sensory and motor functions.

VIII. vestibulocochlear nerve has sensory functions associated with hearing and balance.

IX. The glossopharyngeal nerve coordinates both motor and sensory functions,

X. The vagus nerve is a very diverse nerve that provides both sensory and motor functions,

XI. The accessory nerve is a motor nerve that controls the muscles in the neck, allowing one to rotate, flex, and extend one's neck and shoulders.

XII. The hypoglossal nerve is responsible for the movement of most of the muscles in the tongue.

Chapter One

The Vagus Nerve

The vagus nerve is known as the longest and most complex of the 12 pairs of cranial nerves and it originates from the brain. It is in charge of the transmission of information to or from the brain to tissues and organs connected in the body.

It was originally cited as "pneumogastric" before the name "vagus", which came from the Latin term which literally means "wandering", was adopted. This is because the vagus nerve has the longest and most diverse pathway around the body and is believed, it "wanders" into tissues and organs in the neck, chest, and abdomen from the brain.

It is the 10th cranial nerve out of the 12 cranial nerves and thus known as the "10th cranial nerve" or "cranial nerve X".

The vagus nerve has sensory nerve cell bodies that come in two bunches, and it serves as a connection between the brainstem (from which it originates) to the body (to which it extends to). It allows the brain to receive information and monitor several of the body's different organic and tissue functions.

The vagus is a mixed nerve that contains parasympathetic fibers carrying somatic and visceral afferents and efferents.

The majority of fibers of the vagus nerve are visceral afferents because of the vast nature of cutting across the thoracic and abdominal cavity and its internal organs such as the heart, lungs, stomach, gut, etc and they have a wide distribution that can pass through the central nervous system (CNS). This passage occurs either through the nucleus of the sole tract or monosynaptically. Aside from stimulation of well-defined reflexes, vagus nerve activation produces the manifestation of potentials recorded from the cerebral cortex, the hippocampus, the thalamus, and the cerebellum.

The terminating part of the vagus nerve is called the spinal accessory nucleus.

Etymology

Vagus is a Latin word that means "wandering". It originates from the same root as vagabond, vagrant, divagation and vague.

The vagus nerve is most times described in singular terms even though it is paired but sometimes the right and left branches together are called off in the plural as vagi (/ ˈveɪdʒaɪ/ VAY-jy).

The vagus was once historically called the pneumogastric nerve since it was known to be in charge of innervating both the lungs and the stomach.

Structure

Originating from the medulla oblongata, the vagus nerve runs between the pyramid (olive) and the inferior cerebellar peduncle, it extends through the jugular foramen, then passes into the carotid sheath which is between the internal carotid artery and the internal jugular vein down to the neck, thorax, and abdomen, where it makes contributions to the innervation of the viscera, extending all the way to the colon. That is the reason why it is the longest and most complex of all 12 cranial nerves.

Aside from giving some output to various organs as efferent functions, the vagus nerve is made up of between 80% to 90% of afferent nerves mostly transmitting sensory information about the state and wellbeing of the body's organs to the central nervous system (CNS).

The vagus nerve comes in pair; the right and the left vagus nerves and they descend from the cranial vault passing through the jugular foramina, into the carotid sheath which is between the internal and external carotid arteries, then extends posterolaterally to the common carotid artery. The cell bodies of the vagal visceral afferent fibers are found bilaterally in the inferior vagus nerve ganglia (nodose ganglia).

The right vagus nerve ascends into the neck between the trachea and esophagus when it gives rise to the right recurrent laryngeal nerve and hooking around the right subclavian artery. The right vagus then passes through the anterior to the right subclavian artery, running through the posterior to the superior vena cava, descends posterior to the right main bronchus, and contributes to the complexity of the cardiac, pulmonary, and esophageal plexuses. Forming the posterior vagal trunk at the lower part of the esophagus and it enters the diaphragm through the esophageal hiatus.

The left vagus nerve goes into the thorax between the left common carotid artery and left subclavian artery and descends on the aortic arch which gives rise to the left recurrent laryngeal nerve, hooking around the aortic arch to the left of the ligamentum arteriosum which then travels upwards in between the esophagus and trachea. Some thoracic cardiac branches then branch from the left vagus and further breaks up into the pulmonary plexus, continuing into the esophageal plexus, and then make an entrance into the abdomen as the anterior part of the vagal trunk in the esophageal hiatus of the diaphragm.

The branches include; Pharyngeal nerve, Superior laryngeal nerve, Inferior cervical cardiac branch, Recurrent laryngeal nerve, Thoracic cardiac branches, Branches to the pulmonary plexus, Branches to the esophageal plexus, Anterior vagal trunk, Posterior vagal trunk, Hering-Breuer reflex in alveoli

The vagus nerves run parallel between the common carotid artery and internal jugular vein inside the carotid sheath.

Note; Plexus is a network of an interwoven mass of nerves, blood vessels, or lymphatic vessels.

Nuclei

The vagus nerve includes structurally long, thin fibers called "axons" which originate from the following four nuclei of the medulla:

1. The dorsal nucleus of the vagus nerve – this sends parasympathetic information to the internal organs that lay across the thoracic and abdominal cavity of the body, especially the gut.

2. The nucleus ambiguous – This gives rise to the brachial efferent motor fibers of the vagus nerve and preganglionic parasympathetic neurons that innervate the heart.

3. The solitary nucleus – which receives afferent taste information and primary afferents from visceral organs.

4. The spinal trigeminal nucleus – which receives sensory information about deep/crude touch, pain, and temperature of the outer ear, the dura of the posterior cranial fossa and the mucosa of the larynx.

Development

The motor functional part of the vagus nerve is gotten from the basal plate of the embryonic medulla oblongata, while the sensory functional part of the vagus nerve is derived from the cranial neural crest.

Functions of the Vagus Nerve

The vagus nerve serves both sensory and motor functions

The vagus nerve is a very diverse nerve. It has both sensory and motor functions, including:

1. communication sensation information between your ear canal and parts of your throat

2. Sending sensory information from organs in the chest and trunk, such as the heart and gut to the brain.

3. Allowing motor control of muscles in the throat

4. Aids swallowing by stimulating the muscles of organs in your chest and trunk, and the movement of food through your digestive tract which is known as peristalsis

5. Providing at the root of your tongue, a sense of taste.

The vagus nerve is the cranial nerve with the longest pathway. The pathway starts in a part of the brainstem known as the medulla and travels from the head down into the abdomen. ,

These functions are well elaborated as follows;

1. It serves as a tool for the communication between the guts and the brain: The vagus nerve stands as a messenger between the gut and the brain. It conveys information from the gut about how the body is feeling to the brain for processing via electric impulses known as "action potentials"

2. It helps in reducing heart rate and blood pressure: The vagus nerve helps in lowering the heart rate due to its connection to the heart.

The vagus nerve has a close relationship with the heart. It is in charge of controlling the heart rate via electrical impulses to specialized cardiac muscle tissue known as the heart's natural pacemaker which is in the right atrium, where "acetylcholine" is released to slow down the pulse.

3. It helps in fear management: The vagus nerve sends to the brain, information from the gut, which is linked to stress, anxiety and fear management. This helps a person recover from a scary or stressful situation when faced or triggered by helping the person maintain calmness.

Best explained by saying that the vagus nerve initiates your body to relax.

When the sympathetic nervous system pours the stress hormone, cortisol, and adrenaline into your body, in the "fight or flight" responses. It is the vagus nerve that releases acetylcholine into the body, telling the body to relax. The tendrils of the vagus nerves extend to many organs and act like fiber-optic cables that send instructions to release enzymes and proteins like prolactin, vasopressin, and oxytocin, which calm you down. Vagus nerve response varies from individual to individual for example; people with a weaker vagus response find it difficult to recover from injury, stress or illness while people with a much stronger vagus response may find it less difficult to recover rapidly.

4. Balancing of the nervous system: The nervous system is made up of two areas; first the sympathetic area which is responsible for the increment of alertness, energy, blood pressure, heart rate and breathing and second, the parasympathetic in which the vagus nerve is heavily involved in, which helps in the decrement of the heart rate blood pressure, and alertness and it also helps with calmness, relaxation, and digestion. Therefore, the vagus nerve aids defecation, urination and sexual arousals. Thereby helping to maintain a balance in the nervous system.

Mind you, even though it helps maintain balance in the nervous system, overstimulation of the vagus nerve can cause loss of consciousness

5. It helps in strengthening memory retainment: When the vagus nerve is stimulated, it releases into the amygdala, the neurotransmitter norepinephrine which helps strengthen memories. This according to research and study, suggests a promising future treatment of conditions like Alzheimer's disease.

6. The vagus nerve prevents and decreases inflammation: The vagus nerve sends anti-inflammatory signals to other parts of the body. Inflammation is a physical condition that is sustained during or after injury or illness and it is normal to have a certain amount of it but too much of inflammation is linked to many serious diseases and conditions, ranging from sepsis to the autoimmune condition rheumatoid arthritis. The vagus nerve gets a signal at the slightest detection of inflammation through its operation with a vast network of fibers stationed all around the body's organs.

In the detection of the incipient inflammation —the presence of a substance called tumor necrosis factor (TNF)— alerts the brain and sends out anti-inflammatory neurotransmitters that regulate the body's immune response.

7. Motor functions: The vagus nerve supplies from the neck down to the second segment of the transverse colon to all the organs (except the adrenal glands). It also controls the following: Muscles of the larynx (vocalization), superior, middle and inferior pharyngeal constrictors, palatoglossus muscle, Cricothyroid muscle levator veli palatini muscle, Salpingopharyngeus muscle, Palatopharyngeus muscle

This proves that the vagus nerve is responsible for such varied functions such as heart rate, swallowing, gastro-intestinal peristalsis, sweating, and quite a few muscle movements in the mouth, including speech coordination via the recurrent laryngeal nerve.

8. The vagus nerves help in the breathing process: The neurotransmitter acetylcholine, which the vagus nerve sends as a signal, informs your lungs to breathe, literally. To stimulate your vagus nerve, you can do that by yoga, meditation, abdominal breathing or holding your breath for four to eight counts.

In summary, the vagus nerve as described before is a vast network of nerves that has a pathway to almost all the body's organs. Due to the connection and the active transmission of information from the brain to the organs or from the organs to the brain aids in the other functions as well; gag reflex, satiation after eating, vomiting and fainting.

Effects of The Vagus Nerve

The vagus nerves have emotional effects in the body as well as physical effects.

1. The overstimulation of the vagus nerve in response to emotional stress can cause the overcompensation of the parasympathetic nervous system function to a strong sympathetic nervous system response linking with stress, which causes "vasovagal syncope" causing the immediate drop of the blood pressure and heart

rate and can cause uneasiness or trembling. During extreme vasovagal syncope, there will be restriction of blood flow to the brain, which leads to a shortage of blood supply to the brain and one loses consciousness in the process. Although, most times, to make the symptoms subside one has to sit or lie down for the necessary amount of time. Vasovagal syncope affects young children and women more than other groups.

2. It can also lead to temporary loss of bladder control under moments of extreme fear. That explains why when a person is faced with extreme situations that cause the person to fear, the person may tremble and even urinate on himself/herself.

Research has proven that women having had complete spinal cord injury can still have orgasms through the vagus nerve, which can go from the uterus and cervix to the brain.

Vagus Nerve Stimulation (VNS)

The results gotten from the rigorous research and study made on the vagus nerve and its functions have birthed vagus nerve stimulation which has been tested through clinical trials holds promises of a future of treatment and cure of serious, incurable disease.

Vagus Nerve Stimulation (VNS) is a medical procedure whereby the vagus nerve is stimulated either manually or by electrical pulses.

This has been used to try and treat a variety of conditions such as epilepsy, depression, rheumatoid arthritis, etc.

According to research, the effectiveness of Vagus Nerve Stimulation (VNS) has consequently been approved to be used in the treatment of epilepsy and mental illness.

Vagus Nerve Stimulation Implantation

This is a medical procedure, performed by a neurosurgeon, usually takes about 45-90 minutes with the patient most commonly under general anesthesia. Like with all surgeries, the patient stands at the little risk of infection which includes inflammation or pain at the incision site, damage to nearby nerves and constriction of nerves.

The medical procedure requires two small incisions for the implantation of the nerves. The first incision is made on the upper left side of the chest where the pulse generator is implanted while the second one is made, on the left side of the lower neck, along a crease of the skin, where the thin, flexible wires (known as lead) that links the vague nerve to the pulse generator can be put in.

This device is a piece of metal that is flat and round and measures about 10-13 mm thick and 4 centimeters (an inch and a half) across. This figure is dependent on the model because new models are much smaller.

The device contains a battery, which is made to last from one to 15 years and when the battery is low, the device is replaced with a less medical procedure which, this time, requires only the opening chest wall incision.

The device usually activated after implantation, most commonly two to four weeks after implantation, although in some cases it may be activated right in the operating room at the time of implantation. The device is usually programmed by the treating neurologist in his or her office with a small hand-held computer, programming wand and programming software. During the programming, the strength and duration of the electrical impulses are programmed although the quantity of stimulation varies according to the case but is usually initiated at a low level and gradually increased to a suitable level for the patient. The device works continuously and is programmed to switch on and shut off for specific programmed periods of time— for example, 25 seconds on and 6 minutes off.

The patients are provided with a Magnet Bracelet (handheld magnet) to control the device at home, workplace or anywhere which must be activated and programmed by the treating neurologist to magnet mode. This works by delivering extra stimulation despise the programmed treatment schedule whenever the magnet is swept over the pulse generator site. To turn the device off, the magnet is held over the pulse generator while the magnet is in position while removing it will continue the stimulation cycle. All this maneuver performed with the magnet can be done by the patient, family members, friends or caregivers. Literally, it works like a remote control.

The Side effects, most commonly related to stimulation, usually improve over time. These may include any of the following:

Hoarseness in the voice, coughing, tickling of the throat and shortness of breath which is the most common but they are usually temporary.

This procedure can be used to treat the following:

1. Epilepsy

Epilepsy is a common condition that affects both ain abnormally and causes frequent unpredicted seizures.

Seizures are unpredictable bursts of electrical activity in the brain that affects how it works, temporarily. They are characterized by a wide range of symptoms.

Epilepsy has no definite age at which it can, but usually, it starts either in childhood or in people over 60. It's most times, lifelong, but can get gradually better over time.

Knowing that the vagus nerve lowers heart rate and blood pressure and causes calmness, therefore, the stimulation of the Vagus Nerve can reduce the severity or even stop seizures.

In the treatment of epilepsy, this involves a small, electrical device that is similar to a pacemaker. Under the general anesthesia, the device (which has a thin wire called lead connecting it to the vagus nerve) is placed on the person's chest which helps to send at regular intervals, electrical impulses throughout the day to the brain via the vagus nerve.

Vagus Nerve Stimulation is proven to be effective although it is faced with side effects:

1. Sore throat

2. Nausea/ Stomach Discomfort

3. Difficulty in swallowing

4. Shortness of breath

5. Change in voice by making it hoarse

6. Slow heart rate.

It is advised to report to your doctor if any of these symptoms start or persist as they may be ways to reduce or stop them.

2. Mental illness

Vagus Nerve Stimulation is used to treat drug-resistant cases of clinical depression and it is found to help in the treatment in the following:

1. Alzheimer's disease: Since vagus nerve helps one to make memories. This stimulation of the vagus nerve can release into the amygdala, neurotransmitter nore-pinephrine which strengthens memories. Thus this holds a promising future of treatment and cure of Alzheimer's disease.

2. Anxiety disorders: The vagus nerve helps in stress, anxiety and fear management. Therefore, Vagus Nerve Stimulation can help in the treatment of anxiety disorders.

3. Rapid cycling bipolar disorder: This is a pattern of frequent, unique episodes in bipolar disorder. In "rapid cycling", a person with bipolar disorder experiences four or more distinct episodes of mania or depression in one year. It can unpredictably occur at any point in the course of bipolar disorder, and can come and go over many years depending on how well the disorder is being treated; it is not necessarily a "permanent". The vagus nerve has been proven to help in improving one's mood. Therefore, the therapy of stimulating the vagus nerve can help in the treatment of this disorder.

3. Inflammation

Inflammation is usually as a reaction to injury or infection. It is a localized physical condition in which part of the body becomes swollen, reddened and often painful. Since it is known that the vagus nerve helps in decreasing inflammation when the vagus nerve sends an anti-inflammatory signal to the part or parts of the body that needs it. It is believed that Vagus Nerve Stimulation can be used in the treatment of inflammation.

Further research and consideration suggest that since the vagus nerve have pathways to almost all organs of the body, that it holds a promising future in the treatment of the following:

1. Inflammation from Crohn's disease, Parkinson's disease, diabetes mellitus, and rheumatoid arthritis.

2. Intractable hiccups

3. Abnormal heart rhythm and heart failure.

Although we were once saying the same thing for rheumatoid arthritis, now vagus nerve stimulation can be used in the treatment of rheumatoid arthritis which helps reduce the symptoms to a significant level with no serious adverse side effects. Thus, it is believed that this procedure will be used, in the nearest future, to treat some serious incurable diseases.

The vagus nerve has the most extensive and diverse nerve of all the 12 cranial nerves. The vagus nerve functions make tremendous contributions to the autonomic nervous system, which is made up of the parasympathetic and sympathetic parts.

The nerve is responsible for certain sensory activities and motor information for movement within the body.

Essentially, it is the longest and most vast network of nerves that links the neck, heart, lungs, and the abdomen to the brain.

Its pharyngeal and laryngeal branches transmit motor impulses to the pharynx and larynx which results in swallowing and vocalization. its cardiac branches act to decrease the heart rate, its bronchial branch acts to result in the constriction of the bronchi and helps us breathe and its esophageal branches stimulate peristalsis and gastrointestinal secretions by controlling the involuntary muscles in the esophagus, stomach, gallbladder, pancreas, and small intestine.

In summary, it is connected to motor functions in the voice box, diaphragm, stomach and heart and sensory functions in the ears and tongue. It is connected to both motor and sensory functions in the sinuses and esophagus.

The terminating part of the vagus nerve is called the spinal accessory nucleus.

There are multiple nervous system functions provided by the vagus nerve and its relationship with other parts of the body.

The stimulation of vagus nerve afferents can reduce monosynaptic reflexes, depress the activity of spinothalamic neurons, and increase the pain threshold. According to the stimulation parameters; vagus afferent nerve stimulation (tested clinically in animals) can produce what is called desynchronization or "electroencephalographic (EEG) synchronization" own in affecting sleep states. The Vagus nerve afferent stimulation can also influence the activity of interictal cortical spikes produced by topical strychnine application, and either attenuate or stop seizures produced by pentylenetetrazol, 3-mercapto propionic acid, maximal electroshock, and topical alumina gel. Although the mechanisms for the antiepileptic effects of the vagus nerve stimulation are not fully understood.. it is believed to relate to effects on the reticular stimulating system. The vagus provides an easily accessible, peripheral pathway to regulate the Central Nervous System functions.

Vagus Nerve Stimulation

This is a medical procedure whereby the vagus nerves are stimulated either manually or electrically using a device known as stimulator is implanted in the body as an attachment to the vagus nerve.

Vagus Nerve Has Created A New Field of Medicine

Vagus Nerve Stimulation (VNS) used to treat inflammation and epilepsy has been proven successful over time with fewer adverse side effects. This has birthed a whole new field in medicine, known as bioelectronics. The use of implants that deliver electric impulses to various body parts, scientists and doctors hope that this brings the hope of the future to treat illness with fewer medications and fewer side effects, to life.

Chapter Two

Secrets of The Vagus Nerve

You probably do not know certain secrets about the vagus nerves. After reading this, you would find this piece informative, entertaining and enlightening. The vagus nerve is named so because just like a vagabond, it wanders all about sending sensory fibers from your brain stem to your splanchnic organs. You should know by now that it is the longest of all cranial nerves and controls your inner nerve center. Has someone ever used the expression 'go with your gut,' or have you used the expression 'gut feeling' without knowing the original meaning? There is a deeper meaning to the term 'gut feeling' that meets the eye. The vagus nerve serves as a direct line between your brain and your viscera, it keeps track and reacts to interoceptive signals - information about what is going on inside your body.

1. It Is The Tenth Cranial Nerve

It passes through the diaphragm, throat, abdomen, facial muscles and inner ear.

2. The Vagus Nerves Helps You Make Memories

Research was carried out at the University of Virginia and the results show that stimulating vagus nerves in rats strengthened their memory. Further studies also show that in humans, stimulating the vagus nerves could be a treatment for conditions like Alzheimer's disease. This action is known to release neurotransmitter norepinephrine into the amygdala which consolidates memories. The amygdala plays an important role in the social and emotional process of the brain, it acts as a great influence on everything pertaining to health and addiction.

3. It is Highly Connected To Your Heart

The nerve in charge of controlling your heart rate is the vagus nerves via electrical impulses to specialized muscle tissue. By measuring the time between your heartbeats, and plotting a chart to represent it, your heart rate variability can then be determined by doctors. This data is very important in giving information about the resilience rate of your heart and vagus nerves.

4. A Leading Cause of Fainting is The Over Stimulation of the Vagus Nerve

if the sight of blood makes you shiver or when you're down with the flu you get irritated, it is not because you're weak, it is rather because you are experiencing vagal syncope. When you are stressed out, your body responds to this stress and this action overstimulates the vagus nerves. This results in your blood pressure and heart rate to drop. When the syncope is extreme, the rate of blood flow to your brain reduces and you may lose consciousness. Syncope is the term used to refer to fainting. It occurs when someone loses consciousness for a short time due to the decrease of blood flowing to the brain. The term, Vasovagal syncope describes a disorder in which the vagus nerve goes into overdrive in response to a stimulus like emotional stress, exposure to heat, or standing for a long period of time. This results in a drastic decrease in one's heart rate and blood pressure. When the blood vessels in your legs dilate, it permits blood to pool there and when enough blood cannot reach the brain, the patient passes out. The cure most times may be to lie down with their feet higher than their heads or to sit with their heads between their knees. This activity helps increase blood flow to the brain so as to prevent loss of consciousness. It can also be controlled by getting a night of good sleep and drinking enough water. Also, avoid standing for a long period of time. Some persons also come up with irritable bowel syndrome experience. You should relax, put your heads down and sit on the seat of the toilet. This helps keep your blood pressure steady.

5. When The Vagus Nerves are Stimulated Electrically, It Reduces Inflammation and May Inhibit It

Kevin Tracey, a Neurosurgeon was the first researcher to prove that stimulating the vagus nerves can reduce inflammation. An experiment of this was carried out in rats and since it turned out successful, the same experiment was replicated in humans. The results for humans were as well surprising. The creation of implants to stimulate the vagus nerves showed a reduction and remission, in arthritis which has no cure but is often treated with harmful drugs, hemorrhagic shock, and other serious inflammatory syndromes.

6. Ear Tickling Therapy Is a Secret For Staying Young

Tickling ear therapy can rebalance the nervous system. The operations of the nervous system can be affected by using a small electric current to tickle the ear. This helps people age in a healthy manner. Scientists at the University of Leeds UK found that a short daily therapy delivered for two weeks led to a better quality of sleep including improved moods. This therapy is called transcutaneous vagus nerve Stimulation. It delivers electric current to the ear which sends signals to the nervous system through the vagus nerve. This study shows that this therapy can slow down an important effect associated with aging. This therapy helps protect people from chronic diseases which are likely to come by as one gets older like high blood pressure and cardiovascular diseases.

7. The Stimulation Of Vagus Nerves Have Created A New Field In Medicine

Motivated by the success of vagal nerve stimulation in the treatment of inflammation and epilepsy, a new field of medicine called bioelectronics has arisen. Bioelectronics med one deals with the study of electronics in the body. Imagine having electronics somewhere in your body which is capable of regulating nerve signals and make symptoms of certain disorders go away. The field of study that studies this is bioelectronics medicine. Researchers and companies have gone into the research of bioelectronics. GlaxoSmithKline a British company has also ventured into this field and is funding about 25 researches on disease biology and neural signaling. Also, startups are finding this field interesting. Bioelectronics uses implants that deliver electronic impulses to various parts of the body. Through this research, scientists and doctors are working towards treating illnesses with fewer medications and fewer side effects.

8. It Translates Between Your Gut and Brain

Your guts use the vagus nerve like a walkie-talkie to communicate to your brain how you feel through electrical impulses known as action potentials. What we call the enteric nervous system (ENS) refers to about 100 million neurons that regulate the flow of blood, motility, and secretion within the digestive tract. Although the ENS communicates with the autonomous nervous system (ANS), it is independent enough to have its own reflex arcs. As a result of this, scientists now refer to the ENS as the 'gut brain.' You have an idea about the gut feeling now right? You would wonder the place of the vagus nerve in all of this. The vagus nerve serves as a bridge between ENS and CNS. It stands in the gap between them.

Quite a significant amount of the vagus nerve extends to the digestive system. Up to 10-20% of the vagus nerve cells that connect to the digestive system sends a command from the brain to control muscles that move food through the gut. The other 80-90% g the neurons carry sensory information from the intestines and stomach to the brain. The communication line between the brain and gastrointestinal tract is called the GUT-BRAIN axis and it is saddled with the responsibility of informing the brain about the status of muscle contraction and the speed of food passage. A study published in the journal of medicine in 2017, found out that the vagus nerve is closely related to the digestive system and that the Stimulation of the nerve can improve irritable bowel syndrome. Research has shown that the brain-gut axis has a twin that is, the bacteria that live in the intestine. This communicates with the brain through the vagus nerves affecting not only food intake but mood and inflammation responses. Most of the researchers carried out are done in either rats or mice but we know that rats have certain similarities with humans.

Most of the information traveling along the vagus nerve is going in the gut-brain direction thereby keeping the CNS abreast with happenings in the brain number two. The gut-to-brain method of communication is vital in the regulation of mood and fear processing.

9. It Initiates How Your Body Responds To Relaxation

When your nervous system stands up to the fight or flight responses - a period of pouring the stress hormone cortisol and adrenaline into your body. The vagus nerve tells your body to relax by releasing acetylcholine. The tendrils of the vagus nerves extend to other organs of the body like the fiber optic cables that send instructions to release enzymes and proteins like vasopressin, oxytocin, and prolactin which calms you down. People with stronger vagus nerves are more likely to recover more quickly after illness, injury or stress.

10. The Vagus Nerves Helps You Breathe

The neurotransmitter called acetylcholine elicited by the vagus nerves tells your lungs to breathe. This is why Botox which is used in cosmetics has the potential to destroy because it interrupts your acetylcholine production. One way to stimulate your vagus nerve is by holding in your breath or practicing abdominal breathing for some seconds.

11. The Vagus Nerves Prevents Inflammation

Inflammation after an injury or illness is normal but excess of it is linked to many diseases and conditions ranging from Sepsis to the autoimmune condition rheumatoid arthritis. The vagus nerve mode of operation is similar to a vast network of fibers stationed like spies around all your organs. When there is an inflammation signal, the presence of cytokines or tumor necrosis factor (TNF) alerts your brain and draws out anti-inflammatory neurotransmitters capable of regulating the body's immune response.

The vagus nerve acts as a check on your immune system and releases hormones and enzymes like oxytocin and acetylcholine. These enzymes improve memory, reduces inflammation and helps you feel relaxed.

The awareness and mastery of the biofeedback of brain-heart breathing through the vagus nerve helps you to access flow-state.

90% of the nerve fibers existing throughout the stomach and intestines connects to the brain through the intestine and vagus nerve. It is known as the gut brain. The gut brain would be subsequently explained fully.

The term 'vagal tone' portrays a healthy and functional immune system. A healthy vagal tone is measured by the heart's responsiveness to changes in the breathing rate. People who have a higher HRV can easily switch from excitement to relaxation to excitement and can easily recover from stress.

12. The Vague Nerve Is The Longest Nerve In The Human Body

The vagus nerve connects our brain to vital organs of our body like the heart, intestines, lungs, stomach, etc. It is a key component of the parasympathetic system. The vagus nerve is responsible for stimulating the human body's activities when it is at rest. It has an influence on your breathing, your digestive function and indeed, your heart rate. All these affect your mental health to a very large extent.

The strength of one's vagus response is called the vagal tone and it is determined by an electrocardiogram. The electrocardiogram measures the heart rate. Whenever you take in oxygen, your heart beats faster so as to hasten the flow of oxygenated blood around your body. Breathing out slows down your heartbeat rate. The more difference in your heart rate during breathing, the higher your vagal tone.

Research has shown that a high vagal tone makes your body regulate blood glucose levels better and reduces the chances of having diabetes stroke and cardiovascular diseases. Low vagal tone is associated with Inflammation. The vagus nerves reset the immune system and stop the production of the protein that triggers inflammation.

The vagus nerve is the queen of the parasympathetic nervous system and so, the more we engage in stimulating activities like deep breathing, we remove the effects of the sympathetic nervous system.

There are a few hacks to your vagal tone. One of the hacks is called the cold thermogenesis. It is the act of taking a cold bath. Just like Tim Ferris recommends, taking a cold bath has a direct effect on your vagal tone. Another hack is putting your face in ice water. In a bid to have your vagal tone, do not stay too long while keeping your face in ice because it may lead to injuries. Another hack is the heart rate variability hack. This is directly related to shaping your vagal tone. It allows you to gain more control of your nervous system more quickly than every other hack you may know of.

The vagus nerves allow for pitch variability in our voice and regulate our gag reflex. The vagus nerve is involved in the signaling of the muscles of the back of the throat and of the larynx to be up and doing.

15% of the information that passes through the autonomic nervous system is parasympathetic. If these things do not function well or are not treated appropriately, it means your vagus nerve is not working well.

Travelling puts our body in so much stress this is because when we go across time zones, our body cannot dictate what time is it and so our body throws off the melatonin responses. When we change our schedules, our bodies do not know whether we are awake or asleep. The vagus nerve does a lot of work during sleep time to help the recovery of the stress that occurred throughout the day.

Digestive dysfunction is a common sign of vagus nerve dysfunction, this is because the vagus nerves largely control the activities of the digestive system.

Chapter Three

How The Vagus Nerves Affect Mental Health

The vagus nerve is an essential component of the parasympathetic nervous system and it oversees a lot of bodily and mental functions like mood, digestion, immune response, and mood. It sends useful information about the state of the inner organs to the brain through afferent fibers. Research shows that stimulating the vagus nerve is a treatment for depression, and post-traumatic stress disorder.

Some psychiatric conditions like mood and anxiety disorders can be relieved by stimulating the vagal afferent fibers in the gut. This is because the monoaminergic brain systems that affect their conditions will be influenced. The vagus nerve starts from the medulla oblongata between the olive and cerebellar peduncles.

Depresssion stands as one of the leading mental health diseases worldwide. In the Czech Republic, the prevalence rate is 1.0% and in the US, it is 16.6%. Depression poses a financial and economic threat to society. The physiological aspect of depression is a complex one comprising of a lot of genetic and biological processes. Research has shown that chronic exposure to inflammatory cytokines can lead to depression. Depression can, therefore, be treated with anti inflammatory agents capable of reducing depressive symptoms. IBD is also a risk factor for mood and anxiety disorders and these psychiatric conditions increase the risk of aggravation of IBD.

The vagus nerve is instrumental in the treatment of post-traumatic stress disorder. Trauma can lead to the development of the anxiety disorder, post-traumatic stress disorder. It is characterized by hypervigilance, social avoidance, nightmares, and social dysfunctions. Symptoms of PTSD can be divided into four. They are cognitive and affective alterations, changes in arousal and reactivity, avoidance behavior and intrusion symptoms. People affected by PTSD live their lives as though they are under a permanent threat. The vague nerve mediates over post-traumatic stress disorders. The vagal control of the heart rate via myelinated vagal fibers varies with respiration. The vagal influence on the heart is quantified by measuring the rhythmic fluctuation in heart rate. Patients with PTSD are known to have a lower 'high-frequency' heart rate. The vagus nerve helps individuals to produce anxiety and fear responses.

A research carried out shows that rats without gut-to-brain communication through the vagus nerve experienced lower levels of inner anxiety but had a difficult time un-learning conditioned fear responses. This means that the rats performed well on typical rodent anxiety measures but their response to auditory-cued fear conditioning went on for a longer period of time when compared to rats that were controlled. These changes in behavior are linked to differences in GABA and noradrenaline in specific areas of the limbic system.

Vagus Nerve Stimulation (VNS) has proved its worth as a therapeutic option in the treatment and resistance of anxiety disorders including PTSD. VNS is known to reduce anxiety in rats and improve anxiety scale in patients suffering from treatment resistant depression.

Research reveals that when the vagus nerve is stimulated, it makes for better memory. The brain tends to bring back memories both pleasant and unpleasant ones. Vagus Stimulation is a proven treatment for Alzheimer's disease.

If the vagus nerve is not healthy, it cannot counterpoise your sympathetic nervous system and reset your immune system and this can lead to a lot of health conditions usually associated with chronic inflammation. Keeping your vagus nerve and your nervous system healthy is key to the overall health and wellness if the human body. A healthy nervous system is equal to healthy mental health and immune system. Keeping your nervous system healthy prevents a lot of diseases associated with the nervous system.

The vagus nerve is involved with making you feel calmer when you are faced with non-threatening eye contact. It also helps one filter background noise so that one can adequately recognize people's voices.

In summary, when people talk about the mind and body connection, they are referring to the vagus nerve's influence on the physical and mental health of humans and how interconnected they are.

Symptoms of Vagus Nerve Dysfunction

Research into vagus nerves shows that there are lots of conditions that are linked or are being investigated for a link to the nerve. The vasovagal response would be experienced by many persons because of over Stimulation of the vagus nerve. This reduces blood pressure, slows down the heart rate, widens the blood vessels in your legs and a host of other symptoms.

Many persons are not aware that their vagus nerves could be dysfunctional. A lot of people have vagus nerve dysfunction but are not aware of it. When you have vagus nerve dysfunction, you can be healthy but your wound takes time to heal. There is no cure for vagus nerve dysfunction which is why you need to learn to live with it. There are common symptoms of vagus verve disorder. They include:

1. Chronic Nausea

You lose appetite for food because everything becomes nauseating. It is common to vomit the little food taken in. When you vomit most times, you discover that the food you took in did not digest. If this goes on for a long period of time, it might be a sign that you have vagus nerve dysfunction.

2. Weight Loss and Weight Gain

Due to the inability to eat well as a result of nausea, you might shed some weight. Also, when your stomach is not digesting enough food as it ought to, you lose basic nutrients that help maintain healthy body weight.

Weight gain could arise as a result of anxiety, depression, and fatigue.

3. Dizziness and Fainting

Vagus Nerve dysfunction does not have a cure but it can be managed. Exercise is a good way to increase the function of the muscle.

4. Heartburn

This is also a symptom of vagus nerve dysfunction especially if it occurs frequently. It is a common symptom of this disease. It is a burning sensation in the chest that happens when acid comes back up from your stomach.

5. Anxiety

Anxiety is a state of mental uneasiness nervousness, obsession or concern about an uncertain event. When you have a recurring feeling of anxiety, it might just be a symptom of a dysfunctional vagus nerve.

6. Chronic Fatigue

This is a condition where the body feels tired every time. This becomes a thing to worry about because when the body is constantly in a state of tiredness even when it has not done any work, it becomes a problem.

7. Depression

The vagus nerve is connected to your brain and whatever affects your brain could lead to depression. When one is always feeling sick, it takes a toll on one's mental health.

Try to see a doctor if all these symptoms become a recurring one especially for more than one week because serious complications could arise over time. It can lead to malnutrition and dehydration because your body would not be receiving the right nutrients.

Role of The Vagus Nerve in Metabolism

Through the tools for differentiating between the functions of afferent and efferent signaling to different organs, it is very visible that subdiaphragmatic vagal afferent fibers, via negative feedback, have a role in the control of meal size. Mechanosensitive vagal afferent terminals within the gastrointestinal tract suppress meal size in response to distension and chemosensitive vagal afferent terminals suppress meal size in response to nutrient type and quantity. The injection of Anterograde tracers into the nodose ganglia have been able to identify different types of vagal afferent terminals in the gastrointestinal tract that supports the conclusion that the stomach is actively involved in meal termination.

The Role of Vagus Nerve in Gut Brain Signalling

When there is food, the enteroendocrine system releases inhibit food intake by releasing anorectic hormones. When there is no food, the diverse enteroendocrine cells provide orexigenic hormones that stimulate food intake. Vagal afferents neuron located in the nodose ganglia express traces of chemoreceptors on their terminals in the gut that sense these hormones and mechanoreceptors that sense distension. These signals are conveyed to the nucleus tractus solitaries in the hindbrain.

The Role of Vagus Nerve in Obesity

The disruption of the vagus nerve is implicated in the short-term control of feeding. Total subdiaphragmatic vagotomy capsaicin or subdiaphragmatic deafferentation alter meal patterns but results in underwhelming effects on body weight and daily food intake. Although the ablation of the vagus nerves leads to an increase in meal size, there is compensation in meal frequency that prevents long-term changes in food intake or body weight. There are limitations to these techniques though. Like earlier said, these approaches do not give a clear cut difference between efferent and afferent signaling which may act in opposition to each other thereby concealing an important effect of one or the other in energy homeostasis. It is worthy of note that none of these approaches target vagal fibers innervating individual organs. Different organs may be sending opposing signals ablating all signals from multiple organs thereby concealing the importance of a specific organ. These techniques also randomly inhibit anorectic and orexigenic signals which may conceal the importance of one signal over another. Despite all the limitations listed above, the lack of perceptible change in body weight in the absence of vagal signaling has led to the view that the vagus nerve is involved in the short-term but not the long-term control of food intake.

Vagal Blockade

A vagal blockade is a situation where electrodes are placed on the anterior and posterior vagal trunks near the esophagogastric junction along with a subcutaneously implanted neuroregulator. Reversible vagal inhibition is achieved by applying kilohertz frequency alternating current directly to the nerve to block localized electrical conduction. In both preclinical and clinical studies, KHFAC has been demonstrated to be safe. In clinical trials, vagal blockade treatment leads to weight loss, earlier satiation during meals and improved glycaemic control and liver function. It also reduces blood pressure in obese subjects.

Vagal blockade promotes weight loss in obese subjects. In a clinical trial of obese subjects, the intermittent vagal blockade (VBLOC) significantly improved symptoms of obesity. VBLOC inhibits both afferent signaling and as demonstrated by altered brain imaging an efferent function indicated by minimal pancreatic secretion and gastric contractions. In diabetic subjects, the use of VBLOC reduced body weight, fasting plasma glucose levels and glucose bound hemoglobin.

Targeting The Vagus Nerve With Pharmacotherapy For The Treatment of Obesity

Because of the increasing evidence, and its situation in a peripheral association that is accessible, the vagus nerve is a trusted pharmacological target for treating obesity. Vagal afferent neurons and their terminals including vagal efferent preganglionic terminals are based outside the blood-brain barrier. The drugs specially designed to target the vagus nerve that is too large to cross the blood-brain barrier could be well effective even without unwanted side effects usually caused by off target interactions at central sites. When disrupted vagal agent signaling is addressed, it has the potential to lead to multifaceted benefits including reducing impulsivity and wanting satiation, and increasing thermogenesis. The plasticity of vagal neurons makes them inherently rewireable, with changes in vagal afferent and efferent neurons having been demonstrated to be changeable.

Currently, there are no pharmacological agents designed to particularly target the vagus nerves but there could be an attractive target site for future drug development. It is worthy to note that although no drug in the market specifically targets the vagus nerves, some of the anti obesity may be working in favor of the vagus nerve. Researches have been carried out on the central mechanisms of anti-obesity drugs; however, it still remains unclear the extent to which their effects on significant weight loss are mediated through a vagal pathway.

Vagotomy

This is the term used to refer to the cutting of the vagus nerves. It a therapy that is now out of date. It was performed for peptic ulcer disease. This process is currently under research because it is seen as a less invasive alternative weight loss procedure for gastric bypass surgery. The gastric bypass surgery is a surgical process where the stomach is divided into a small pouch and a larger pouch and the small intestine is rearranged to connect both the small and large pouch. Gastric bypass surgery leads to a reduction in the functional volume of the stomach accompanied by an alteration in the physiological and physical response to food. This procedure is carried out in obese patients to reduce the feeling of hunger and it is performed by putting bands on the patient's stomach resulting in the patient losing about 43%of excess weight after six months of healthy diet and exercise. The vagotomy procedure does not come without side effects. One side effect common in vagotomy patients is the vitamin B12 deficiency about ten years after the procedure. This is similar to pernicious anemia (it is a disease where there is a reduction in the production of red blood cells due to the deficiency of vitamin B12). The vagus normally stimulates the stomach's parietal cells to secrete acid and intrinsic factor. The intrinsic factor is vital in the absorption of vitamin B12 from food. A vagotomy reduces the secretion of Vitamin B12 which ultimately leads to the deficiency which If left untreated, it may lead to nerve damage, paranoia, dementia and eventually death. Research done in the Aarhus University and Aarhus University hospital show that vagotomy prevents the development of Parkinson's disease (a long time degeneration of the central nervous system that affects the motor system). This research suggests that Parkinson's disease begins in the gastrointestinal tract and spreads from the vagus nerve to the brain. In summary, vagotomy is a surgical procedure that removes part of the vagus nerve and serves numerous functions in the body like controlling the production of stomach acid. These days, the vagotomy procedure is done side by side with other procedures. Recent research has shown that the vagotomy procedure is more advantageous than doctors thought.

The Vagus Nerve and Digestion

When the function of the vagus nerve is disrupted, digestion also would be disrupted. Symptoms range from heartburn or inflammatory bowel disease like ulcerative colitis and it is capable of preventing the body from healing small intestine bacteria overgrowth. A consistent cause of Irritable Bowel Syndrome. The vagus nerve is one of the systems that tell the stomach to put out all the digestive acids and juices and start the movement of the gut. When we chew our food in our mouth, we start the process of mixing in your food with digestive acids and enzymes that begin the process of breaking down food before it reaches our stomach and then to the small and large intestine. If the vagus nerve does not send the right signal, the flow of food mixed with acid through the gut is slowed. This means that there would be an overgrowth of bacteria, yeast or parasites as well as hormones and toxins that are not used up, the ones the body works very hard to eliminate. The risk of IBS and SIBO is increased when there is higher exposure to bacteria, waste products and thus worsens any infections present. When your body is exposed to more hormones than your body can accommodate, hormonal imbalance occurs.

Vagus Nerve, MMC And SIBO

MMC means migrating motor complex and SIBO means Small intestine bacterial overgrowth. The MMC can be likened to the caboose of a little train moving through our intestines. When you eat, the food that is chewed combines with digestive acids and enzymes and is loaded on the train to be moved out of your body in the form of stool. There are so many factors capable of stopping the train, a reduced vagus nerve firing is one of the major contributors to MMC dysregulation. The train ought to move through the central station, that is, the place after your stomach and then to the final stop which is the anus. This trip ought to be a one-way trip, so much so that the train should leave the station and reach the end of the road every 90-120 minutes. Whenever you eat, the train stops and goes backward in order to pick a new food passenger showing the movement of food through your digestive tract which can result in bacterial overgrowth and increased toxin burden in the body. The MMC could also be confused or misguided by stress, trauma, and other life factors.

Foods That Can Calm Your Vagus Nerve

Most persons have busy days characterized by early morning juggling, rushing out early so as to beat traffic, engaging in one activity or another just to make ends meet. As a result of these activities, our stress hormones are activated and managing stress is somewhat impossible for some persons. When there is high cortisol, it is very dangerous to the body. One of the dangers is that it triggers food craving which may leave you craving for a box of chocolate and ice cream. This same cortisol can make an enzyme in the body transform cortisone into even much more cortisol. Certain foods can restore the calm our life needs. It is not the kind of food that gives temporary relief but the ones that proffer permanent solution. To say the truth, there is always a feeling of guilt when you take in a pint of ice cream or any snack. There are foods with the ability to calm your vagus nerves because of their nutritional content like foliate which is a stress reducer and energy giver. There are foods that are capable of relieving stress and restore internal equilibrium. You would not regret including these foods in your diet. The foods are as follows:

Asparagus

This food is rich in foliate. A study carried out in over 2,600 adults found out that people who ate foods rich in foliate are at a much more reduced risk of having depression than those who consumed a lesser amount.

Avocados contain more foliate than any other fruit and they contain healthy fats and potent antioxidants like glutathione, beta carotene, vitamin E, and lutein which is capable of fighting cell-damaging free radicals. They are slightly high in calories and so, you do not need to consume it in hight quantity before it acts on your nerves.

Berries

Berries are a source of vitamin C which is known from time immemorial to reduce stress. In a double-blind, placebo-controlled study, about 500 milligrams of vitamin C was found to reduce anxiety among high school students. A separate study also found out that vitamin C was instrumental in the reduction of anxiety among patients with type two diabetes.

Chamomile Tea

This tea is surely a tested and trusted way to calm your nerves. Two separate studies from the University of Pennsylvania further buttress this fact. In the first study conducted in 2009, 57 adults with anxiety and depression problems were given Chamomile extract for eight weeks and there was a clear difference after eight weeks. There was an improvement in the lives of those persons that took the Chamomile tea and those that didn't take it remained the same. Another follow-up study conducted in 2012 also showed that chamomile provided an antidepressant benefit along with reducing anxiety. Chamomile tea is prepared by pouring 8 ounces of boiling water over 2 or three tablespoons of dried chamomile and soak for about 10 minutes. It can be served over ice too.

Dark Chocolate

Chocolate naturally offers a sense of relief. Dark chocolate is absolutely more than just food but it can boost serotonin levels as well as reduce blood pressure and provide a sufficient amount of antioxidants in the form of polyphenols and flavonols. In any case, moderation is key in the intake of chocolates. In as much as chocolates boost the production of serotonin, taking chocolates in large quantities is dangerous to the health.

Fermented Foods

There is a direct connection between the brain and guts as we know. Fermented foods contain sources of bacteria called probiotics and this has a direct impact on the chemistry of the brain through your vagus nerve. A 2016 review study from Canada noted the psychological benefits of this probiotics supplementation. In making your selection for food, ensure to verify the number of probiotics. You can even make your own fermented veggies, kefir, sauerkraut, and yogurt.

Fish

Consuming omega 3 fatty acids increases vagal tone, says research. It also puts you into a calming parasympathetic mood.

Leafy Greens

Leafy greens like Kale, spinach, Swiss chard, mustard greens, and many other leafy greens are a good source of folate and magnesium which is another vital nutrient capable of calming the nerves. A meal with asparagus, some slices of avocado and leafy greens are the meal your nerves would be thankful for.

Seeds

Seeds like flax, hemp, chia, sesame seeds contain a sufficient amount of magnesium which is one of the compounds that participates in the chemical reaction of serotonin. Deficiency in magnesium can lead to anxiety, depression, and all forms of panic attack. A study shows that taking magnesium is associated with reduced symptoms of depression. Another study carried out in 5,708 adults showed that there is a relationship between the intake of magnesium and depression.

Oatmeal

Oatmeal reduces stress in two ways. Oatmeal is affordable and easy to make. A plate of oatmeal could be garnished with berries for a sumptuous meal.

Diet is very important when it comes to improving our vagus nerves. Carefree eating does not help the brain, the nervous system and the vagus nerve particularly.

Circadian Rhythm

A modern problem that occurs on a daily basis is circadian rhythm or the natural sleeping and waking rhythm of our bodies. Part of this problem is that most persons hardly engage in active work during the day. They do not walk, rather they take a car to their destination, sit for 8-10 hours and do not exercise their body. Then at night, we are glued to our phones, tablets, television, and computers. The light from our phones communicates to our brains that it is time to be awake. This is a tempting sight to behold because the temptation to check social media before going to bed would always be there. Reading a book before going to bed is a more profitable venture. The vagus nerve transmits the signal from the circadian control center in the brain. Effects of circadian dysregulation is bi-directional. When the circadian flow is interrupted, it affects the brain and it changes the hormone levels and melatonin and this can lead to problems with the vagus nerve which in the long run affects the rest of your body. Also, the circadian control center in your brain also sends a signal to the digestive system and lungs which produces mucin - the substance that keeps your organ healthy and well lubricated.

Drug Development For The Vagus Nerve

An advantage of developing drugs that target the vagus nerve is it's preventing of brain penetration. It could reduce the severity of side effects by reducing off-target effects of unwanted binding at central sites. Theoretically, this enables the use of a higher dose or a combination of multiple therapies. However, restricting just one drug to the outside alone is not sufficient to ensure that there are no side effects. A drug could have off-target effects by interacting with visceral organs but the vagus nerve modulates a lot of physiological functions like cardiorespiratory control. The important challenge will be to selectively target drugs to vagal afferents innervating abdominal organs thereby drastically reducing the risk of cardiorespiratory side effects. A possible mechanism used to achieve cell type specificity includes developing antibody drug conjugates similar to those used by chemotherapy drugs to target cancerous cells. In a case like this, the antibody binds a receptor expressed on vagal afferent neurons innervating the gut and presents a miming hormone that agonizes or antagonizes a second receptor.

An important question in designing drugs that target the vagus nerve is whether the drug would only be effective when binding at afferent terminals or whether binding to the cell bodies and a on produces a similar effect. However, a drug that is taken orally and absorbed by the small intestine would activate vagal afferent terminals and when taken at a higher dose, it could activate the neuronal bodies in the nodose ganglia.

The Relationship Between Parkinson's Disease and The Vagus Nerve

An experiment carried out at John Hopkins University using mice, discovered that Parkinson's disease originates among cells in the guts and travels through the vagus nerve to the brain. This study offers a new and accurate model to test treatment that can prevent Parkinson's disease progression. The findings provide proof of the role of the gut in Parkinson's disease and gives a model to study the disease from the beginning.

Parkinson's disease is identified by a build-up of mis-folded protein known as alpha-synuclein, domiciled in the cells of the brain. When these proteins continue to gather together, they cause the tissue of the nerve to die off leaving large lumps of dead brain matter known as Lewy bodies. As time goes on, these brain cells die thereby impairing a person's ability to move, think or control emotions. This new study builds on the obser-vations made in 2003 by a neuroanatomist Heiko Braak which showed that people with Parkinson's dis-ease had an accumulation of misfolded alpha-synu-clein protein in some parts of their central nervous sys-tem that controls the gut. The appearance of these pro-teins that damage the nervous system are consistent with some symptoms of Parkinson's disease like con-stipation.

Another evidence has speculated that the gut-brain has a connection in initiating the Parkinson's disease. The researchers were curious as to whether the alpha-synu-clein is capable of traveling along the vagus nerve which runs like an electric cable from the stomach and small intestine up to the brain. To test the validity of this, researchers injected 25 mg of synthetic misfolded alpha-synuclein created in the lab into about a dozen healthy mice. They sampled and analyzed the tissue af-ter one month, three months, seven months and ten months after introducing the injection. As the experiment progressed, the researchers found out that the alpha-synuclein began to form close to the vagus nerve connected to the gut and gradually spread to all parts of the brain.

Similar research was carried out soon after but this time with a different method. This time, the vagus nerve in a group of mice was surgically cut off and their guts were injected with misfolded alpha-synuclein. After seven months, the researchers found out that the mouse with severed vagus nerves showed no signs of cell death as opposed to mouse with their vagus nerve intact. When these nerves are severed, they halt the advances of misfolded protein advancing beyond normal. They also investigated whether the physical differences in Parkinson's disease results in behavioral changes. To carry out this investigation, they studied the behavior of three groups: mice injected with misfolded alpha-synuclein, mice injected with misfolded alpha-synuclein and cut vagus nerves and mice with no injection and an intact vagus nerves. They focused on tasks they use to distinguish signs of Parkinson's disease in mouse-like nest building or exploring a new environment.

The researchers observed that the mice built nests in their domain and this is usually a characteristic of Parkinson's disease in humans. Seven months after the injection, the researchers provided nesting materials for the mice and watched their behavior for about 16 hours scoring them on a scale of 0-6. They discovered that Mice that received the misfolded alpha-synuclein injection scored low in terms of nest building.

The mice with severed vagus nerves scored 3 to 4 on a scale of 0 to 6. The mice that received the misfolded alpha-synuclein scored lower than 1. Also, the group of mice that received the alpha-synuclein used an infinitesimal amount of nesting material (less than one gram).

In summary, the result of this study shows that misfolded alpha-synuclein is transferable from the gut to the brain in mice alongside the vagus nerve and if the transmission route is blocked, it prevents the physical and cognitive manifestations of Parkinson's disease. Researches say they would venture into another research to find out the part of the vagus nerve that allows the misfolded protein to climb the brain and also investigate ways it can be stopped.

Chapter Four

The Vagus Nerve and Anxiety

Including all the wonderful things the vagus nerve does in the body such as contributing to the sensitivity of the respiratory mucous membranes and transmitting the rhythm, as well as intervening in the transmission of strength and frequency of breathing, the vagus nerve equally receives signals from the internal organs and sends them to the brain to be processed. The signals sent to the brain are also sent around the body through motor neurons and transmitters. The motor neurons and transmitters are the things that tell other parts of the body to carry out an activity or not to.

The signals sent from the brain across the body are responsible for various emotions such as nervousness, calmness and anger. Such process of transmission of signals shows that there is a relationship between the vagus nerve and anxiety. Hence, for you to fully capture the relationship between the vagus nerve and anxiety you need to comprehend the activities of the two contrasting systems that are always sending information to the brain.

One of the two opposite systems is the sympathetic nervous system. Its job is to prepare you for action, by supplying your body with the right quantity of adrenaline and cortisol. These hormones are responsible for the quickening of the heart rate and general body alertness when there is a need to act on an impulse, albeit spontaneously. And when you have acted on the needed action, the other system – the parasympathetic nervous system – will work to ensure your body returns to a state of homeostasis; which is a state of rest and calmness.

The job of both systems is to accelerate and decelerate body feelings and emotions. When your body is high-up on adrenaline, the parasympathetic nervous system decelerates you to a state of relaxation. The acceleration and deceleration process uses acetylcholine, a neurotransmitter that decreases the heart rate and blood pressure in order to enable the organs to work faster, and this does not happen without the full integration of the vagus nerve.

The vagus nerve has tons of roles it plays in the body. Being that it is the tenth out of twelve pairs of the cranial nerves, the vagus nerve is the longest of all nerves in the body; snaking its way from the cranial box in the spinal cord through the neck where it develops into two branches, and then down to the abdomen where it passes through all the organs located along its path.

The functions of the vagus nerve in relation to anxiety

The vagus nerve is in control of the parasympathetic system, and it takes part in many functions such as mouth movement and heartbeat. But when it's affected by other factors, it can trigger some symptoms such as anxiety. The functions of the vagus nerve in relation to anxiety are:

-Heartbeat regulation, controlled muscle movements, and regulated breathing.

It is actively involved in maintaining the functionality of the digestive tract, thereby making it possible for the muscles in the stomach and intestine to digest food.

It is equally responsible for facilitating relaxation after a stressful event, and likewise, it triggers the feeling that there is danger, thereby keeping you alert through-out the period the feeling lasts. It is responsible for sending sensory information to the brain with regard to the status of other organs.

Having discussed the salient functions of the vagus nerve in relation to anxiety and what goes on in the body between the vagus nerve and other organs that might be affected during an anxiety episode, the rela-tionship of the vagus nerve and anxiety and how the latter affects the former would be discussed.

-How anxiety affects the vagus nerve:

The sympathetic nervous system is usually activated whenever you experience any stressful event. If the stress persists over a longer period of time and there isn't just a way the psychological response that trig-gered it could be effectively addressed, the prolonged period of tension would birth a lot of emotional and mental problems. When the period of stress is on-going, dual-pathway activation is opened in the brain: the hypothalamus – pituitary – adrenal pathway and the brain – intestine pathway.

This is how it works. Normally, the brain responds to anxiety and stress by increasing the production of some hormones (CFRs), which travel all the way from the hypothalamus to the pituitary gland where they assemble to enhance the release of another hormone which will in turn travel through the bloodstream to the adrenal glands. When the hormone (ACTH) reaches the adrenal glands it will stimulate the integration of adrenaline and cortisol. These hormones (adrenaline and cortisol) when activated suppress the immune system and influence inflammation in the body. These activities are the reason some certain things happen, which could be the reason why you get the feeling that you're ill whenever you are stressed or you're anxious over a thing. But when this feeling is not handled it can lead to depression. Depression as a disorder is often linked to an inflammation in brain response.

You should know that there is a high tendency for there to be an increase in glutamate in the brain caused by chronic stress and prolonged anxiety. Glutamate is a neurotransmitter that the excess production of it causes migraine, depressions and anxiety disorder. And when you are tensed, stressed and always anxious, there is a possibility that you will have so much deposit of cortisol in your blood. Cortisol, when there is a high level of it in the blood, leads to the reduction in the volume of hippocampus. Hippocampus is the part of the brain that is responsible for the formation of new memories. This means that there will be a high level of restlessness in the body, and all these have a way of affecting the vagus nerve.

When the vagus nerve is affected by conditions such as the one mentioned above, symptoms like dizziness, gastrointestinal conditions, arrhythmias, difficulty in breathing, and a host of negative emotional responses will manifest. And the condition will prevent the vagus nerve from initiating a state of relaxation or the signal that will initiate it. When this happens, the sympathetic nervous system will keep functioning, causing every action and response to be impulsive. What this shows on its own part is the beginning of anxiety.

There are times when one could be born with negative impulsiveness as a congenital ailment. This is mostly as a result of poor vagal tone during pregnancy. A study carried out in the University of Miami discovered that women who were mostly anxious and depressed for the better part of their pregnancy are likely to transmit there poor vagal tone to their fetus. When this happens the children when born would likely exhibit low vagal activity, and would most like secrete lower levels of dopamine and serotonin.

Chapter Five

Vagus Nerve Stimulation

In stimulating the vagus nerve, there is a process known as the vagal response. This simply means a stimulation of the vagus nerve. Vagal response and vagal tone are implicated with each other. The vagal tone is a biological process that encompasses all the activities of the vagus nerve. The vagus nerve runs through all your internal organs. Whenever the parasympathetic nervous system is activated, it means there is an increase in vagal tone. And when this happens it becomes possible for you to relax very well after a stressful day or activity. Your ability to relax makes it all possible for your health to improve generally, and your systems working affectively.

Vagus nerve stimulation is precisely a particular method of medical treatment employed by a physician during the treatment of epilepsy and any other of the numerous neurological health conditions. This is how the stimulation works. It is achieved by applying electrical impulses on the vagus nerve, and this stimulation works in two particular ways: the direct invasive stimulation and the indirect transcutaneous non-invasive stimulation. Currently, the direct invasive stimulation is the frequently most used application. Both major and minor invasive vagus nerve stimulation (iVNS) is carried out through implanting a small pulse generator subcutaneously in the left thoracic region via a surgical process.

When this is done, electrodes that are connected to pulse generator by a lead, which is also tunneled under a skin are then attached to the left cervical vagus nerve. At this point the work of the generator is to deliver intermittent electrical impulses through the vagus nerve to the brain. The understanding is that these electrical impulses exist to exert antidepressive, anti-inflammatory, and antiepileptic effects by changing the excitability of nerve cells.

But in all these there is a case. As a contrast to invasive vagus nerve stimulation, transcutaneous vagus nerve stimulation gives room for the non-invasive stimulation of the vagus nerve without the assistance of any surgical procedure. And for this to happen, the stimulator is often attached to the auricular concha through ear clips, while delivering electrical impulses at the subcutaneous course of the afferent auricular branch of the vagus nerve.

In an article by Sackeim HA et al titled "Vagus nerve stimulation (VNStm) for treatment-resistant depression: efficacy, side effects, and predictors of outcome," a pilot study was done when there was an examination of the application of VNS in sixty patients who has treatment-resistant depressive disorder. It showed that there was a significant clinical improvement in about 30-37% of the patients, recording a higher level of tolerability. Some years later, following the discovery of the pilot study, the stimulation of the refractory depression was approved by the United States Food and Drug Administration (FDA). That was a pivotal moment in medicine. Beginning from that time, the safety and efficacy of vagus nerve stimulation in the case of any major depressive disorder has been made a part of tons of observational studies.

The Neural Mechanism of Vagus Nerve Stimulation

The research work done by Chae J-H et al titled "A review of functional neuroimaging studies of vagus nerve stimulation (VNS)," covers a lot of ground as regards vagus nerve stimulation and the neurology behind it. According to information obtained from the work mentioned above, functional neuroimaging studies have certainly confirmed that vagus nerve stimulation changes the activity of a lot of cortical and subcortical regions. This is done through direct or indirect anatomic connections through the NTS. This is because the vagus nerve has structural connections and links with many of the mood regulating limbic and cortical brain areas, which means that in an instance of chronic vagus nerve stimulation for depression, PET scans will most likely show a decline in the possibility of resting brain activity in the ventromedial prefrontal cortex (vmPFC). The decline also projects to the amygdala and some other brain regions responsible for regulating emotion.

Oftentimes, vagus nerve stimulation results in chemical changes that occur in monoamine metabolism in these regions, which also has the tendency to result in antidepressant action. The relationship that exists in the action that occurs between monoamine and antidepressant has been captured by different types of evidence, which conclude that all the drugs that increase monoamines – serotonin (5-HT), NE, or dopamine (DA) – within the synaptic cleft often contains antidepressant properties. This refers to the danger of an increased risk of depression caused by a depletion of monoamines which in turn induces depressive symptoms in individuals who are prone to depression.

Carpenter LL, et al, in their research work titled: "Effects of vagus nerve stimulation on cerebrospinal fluid monoamine metabolites, norepinephrine, and gamma-aminobutyric acid concentrations in depressed patients," said that "chronic vagus nerve stimulation influences the concentration of 5-HT, NE, and DA in the brain and in the cerebrospinal fluid," which means that chronic vagus nerve stimulation is usually associated with increased extracellular levels of serotonin in the dorsal raphe.

How to Stimulate the Vagus Nerve to Enhance Mental wellness

Developing a sharp and complete understanding of how your vagus nerve works will make it much easier for you to work with your nervous system instead of feeling subdued when it seems to work against you. Being the longest nerve in the body and connecting the brain to many important organs and systems throughout the body, the vagus nerve plays a key role in the activities of the parasympathetic nervous system. It also coordinates and influences the pattern, quality and frequency of breathing, the level of digestive function, and heart rate. All these have precise impact on your mental wellness, and if you want to maximize the benefit, you need to stimulate your vagus nerve.

To stimulate your vagus nerve, you need to pay attention to your vagal tone. Your vagal tone is the ability of your body to return to a state of homeostasis after a period of stress. When you increase your vagal tone, your parasympathetic nervous system would be activated. Stimulating your vagal tone increases the activities of the "feel good hormone," thereby ensuring you have a good physical and mental health. Vagus nerve stimulation reduces stress; it keeps the heart rate and blood pressure at optimal level, and it stimulates digestion. The benefits are numerous, but before you know what the benefits are you should know how to stimulate it. To stimulate the vagus nerve, you should consider doing the following:

Expose yourself to cold a little bit. Studies have revealed that exposure to cold activates the vagus nerve and also activate the cholinergic neurons through the vagus nerve pathway. This works to lower your sympathetic response to stress (that's the fight or flight response), and at the same time increase parasympathetic activities through the vagus nerve (that's the ability to enter a complete state of relaxation after a stressful event or an episode of anxiety). To do achieve this kind of vagal activity, you might have to consider taking cold showers and walking the length and breadth of your front pouch with minimal clothing during cold temperatures (now this does not in any way signify any unreasonable exposure to cold). You can also try making the last part of your shower period a cold bath (say the last thirty to forty seconds of your shower period should be completed with cold water). Or you can try a more subtle way by sticking your face into a bowl of ice-cold water. If you are hypertensive, or have suffered a previous heart attack, you might have to consult with your doctor before you do this. You don't have to shock your brain unexpectedly with cold water. Refrain from pouring cold water directly on your head. The idea is to enhance your vagal tone, and not to cause any damage to your health.

Practice deep and slow breathing. Some people inhale air for about fourteen to fifteen times within a minute. This indicates that their breathing is shallow and quick. But it shouldn't be so. You should aim to inhale air at most seven times in every minute. Inhaling air within longer and deeper periods has been proved to stimulate the vagus nerve, reduce anxiety, relieve stress and increase the activities of the parasympathetic nervous system. When you breathe, it should be deep and longer, and when you exhale it should equally be long and slow. This way your stomach will expand outward, air will be transported to the lower part of your chest, and your vagus nerve will be adequately stimulated.

You should sing, hum, gargle and chant. The vagus nerve is connected to the vocal cords and to the muscles at the back of the throat. Hence, when you do the above, the muscles controlling these activities would be activated, and likewise your vagus nerve would be stimulated. These activities have also been proved to increase heart-rate variability and the attendant vagal tone.

Meditate at regular intervals. Meditation is a fine relaxation technique that has a wider tendency to stimulate the vagus nerve and also increase vagal tone. It increases positive emotions and also promotes the feelings of goodness towards oneself and a general feeling of wellness. It also reduces the effect of the activities of the sympathetic nervous systems such as the fight or flight response, but increases vagal modulation.

You can also practice activities such as Yoga and Tai Chi. These are important mind-body relaxation techniques that work by stimulating your vagus nerve and enhancing the activities of your parasympathetic nervous system. It is essential you practice it because it is helps you relax during periods of anxiety and depression. According to a study carried out at Boston University, yoga should be integrated in every day routine, because it increases the GABA neurotransmitters, which are held to be responsible for the promotion of the feeling of calm and serenity, and thereby helping in combating stress and anxiety. Whereas tai-chi is known for its ability in helping to balance heart rate. When there is a feeling of calm and serenity and the heart rate is balanced, it means that there is stimulation in vagal modulation. Hence, these activities are ideal for stimulating the vagus nerve.

Learn to consume omega-3 fatty acids. These are essential fats your body cannot produce by itself, but which your body desperately needs. These fatty acids are primarily derived from fish, and they are necessary for the normal electrical functioning of your brain and nervous system. Omega-3 fatty acids are indispensable when it concerns mental health, and they also concern several other aspects of wellness. Numerous researches have shown that omega-3 fatty acids enhance vagal tone; they reduce heart palpitation, but increases heart rate variability, which in turn means that they have the tendency to stimulate the vagus nerve. Consuming fish and other omega-3 fatty acids supplement will improve vagus nerve stimulation.

Exercising regularly has the tendency to enhance the growth of your brain's hormones, it will support brain's mitochondria, and will help reverse cognitive decline. If you want to experience the manifestation of these, try stimulating your vagus nerve through exercise. You could engage in mild and not-too-rigorous exercise. Exercises like lifting heavy weights, sprinting, and power-walk are all good forms of exercise that are capable of stimulating the vagus nerve.

Have yourself massaged at intervals is enough to increase vagal tone and also stimulate your vagus nerve. You can achieve this by massaging specific areas of your body, like foot massage. Foot massages also known as reflexology have proved to increase heart rate variability. It also helps with vagal modulation. When you massage the area around the right side of your throat known as the carotid sinus, the activity can stimulate the vagus nerve to reduce seizures in a case of epilepsy or the likes of it.

Laughing heartily is also another means of stimulating your vagus nerve. It will decrease your body's main stress hormone, but increase positive emotions. It has been proven that laughter has the potential to increase heart-rate variability, and the vagus nerve stimulation often comes with laughter as the side benefit.

Acupuncture is an alternative treatment that has proved to help in stimulating the vagus nerve. It works faster for people who are about rounding off their mental health treatment, especially those who are on anti-depressants. It has been proven that ear acupuncture stimulates the vagus nerve; thereby increasing vagal activity and tone, and can also help in the treatment of neurodegenerative diseases such as schizophrenia and any of the acute phobias. This kind of treatment can be conducted through vagal regulation.

You have seen the ways your vagus nerve can be stimulated. It has also been discussed how beneficial a well-stimulated vagus nerve is, which is to reduce stress and heart rate coupled with blood pressure. It also affects the functioning of some certain parts of the brain, helps in stimulating digestion, and all the other nice things the body does or initiates when it is at rest. But this is not all there are to what the vagus nerve can do. Studies have shown that stimulating the vagus nerve and the attendant increased vagal tone are affective when it comes to treating a variety of mental and health conditions such as:

- Depression.
- Alzheimer's disease.
- Migraine.
- Anxiety disorders.
- Fibromyalgia.
- Tinnitus.
- Addictions (any of the substance abuse).
- Autism.
- Any of the eating and personality disorders.
- Amnesia.

- Dementia and mood disorders in older people.

- Obsessive compulsive disorder and post traumatic stress disorder.

- Severe mental diseases and any traumatic brain injury.

- Chronic fatigue syndrome, social phobias, and insomnia.

While the stimulation of the vagus nerve proves to be effective in the treatment of the above ailments, it might also interest you to know that stimulating the vagus nerve can equally reduce inflammation in the body just the way it helps with the other health conditions. The following chapter would be devoted to discussing how stimulating the vagus nerve reduces inflammation and the symptoms of arthritis.

Chapter Six

Vagus Nerve Stimulation to Reduce Inflammatory Responses

Inflammatory response occurs when tissues get infected or harmed by bacteria, toxins, trauma, heat, or any other cause. Inflammatory response is the reason excessive heat causes meningitis. It occurs when the damaged cells release chemicals such as prostaglandins, bradykinin, and histamine. These chemicals when released cause the blood vessels to pass fluid into the tissues. The leaked fluid into a place it shouldn't be is the reason for swelling. Though the chemicals works to help heal the wound by alerting the body of the presence of an unusual occurrence, there are other times the inflammation they create plays a role in the appearance of chronic diseases such as heart diseases or stroke, and could lead to the development of autoimmune disorders such as lupus, rheumatoid and arthritis. This happens when the inflammation stays on for too long in the body and begins to form plaques in the blood.

Having seen how inflammation develops and how disturbing its presence could be, it is important you understand how its responses play key roles in the development and persistence of many diseases in the body; diseases that can lead to a weakening chronic pain. There are other times inflammation could be a body's response to stress. Hence, when you experience the kind of pain and weakness inflammation causes, if you could reduce the happenstance of stressors that lead to the release of cortisol, and thereby reducing the regularity of the fight or flight response in your sympathetic nervous system, such reduction will most likely reduce inflammation caused by stress.

There are some medical prescriptions built to combat inflammation and its attendant risks. Nonetheless, there is an established way to combat inflammation by incorporating the vagus nerve. This will make use of other forms of vagal responses chief among them is the vagal tone. This will not only take care of the inflammation from its root cause, it will also improve the individual's vagal tone. And to do this, healthy daily activities would have to be cultivated. Such daily activities include yoga, Tai Chi and meditations, but if it in an extreme case such as rheumatoid arthritis (RA), treatment could be initiated by implanting a device designed to stimulate the vagus nerve.

Sometime in 1921, a certain German physiologist by the name Otto Loewi made an outstanding discovery. He found out that when the vagus nerve was stimulated, there was a reduction in the heart rate which triggered a kind of substance that did the work of a neurotransmitter. He called the triggered substance "Vagusstoff", which is a German word for vagus substance. The substance was later identified to be acetylcholine, which was the first neurotransmitter to be identified by scientists.

The neurotransmitter acetylcholine functions like a tranquilizer, which could be self-administered by taking in deep breathes. Without having to sound repetitive, you have been told how to breathe and how the right way to breathe contributes in vagal tone. Instead of inhaling air about fifteen to sixteen times per minute, you should do so in longer and deeper intakes for six to seven times. When you do this you have willfully tapped into the state of calmness and relaxation your vagus nerve creates. This activity on its part will take care of your inflammation reflex, because a healthy vagal tone is a sort of a feedback process linked to positive emotions. Hence, when your body is in a state of relaxation, the chances of developing stress-induced inflammation will be reduced, drastically. And there wouldn't be any way prolonged inflammation in the body will lead to the development of chronic diseases such as rheumatoid arthritis.

Vagal Tone Index

A single process indicates the vagal tone, and that is the increase and decrease of heart rate during air inhalation. Healthy vagal tone is indicated by a little increase in heart rate when you breathe in, while it records a decrease in heart rate when you breathe out. And for the vagal response to be complete, you are required to take deep diaphragmatic breathing. This will ensure a good vagal tone and your vagus nerve would be adequately stimulated. Hence, when you record a higher vagal tone index it means you are physically and psychological healthy, while a low vagal tone index is linked to inflammation, depression, anxiety, negative emotions, and cardiovascular problems. Thus, a high vagal tone index could be summarily defined as part of a feedback loop occurring between positive emotions, physical and mental health, and adequate positive social relations.

The Role of Vagus Nerve Stimulation in Reducing Arthritic Inflammation

A research team comprising researchers from the United States and those from Amsterdam conducted a clinical trial which was anchored on stimulating the vagus nerve with a small implanted device. The process is known as invasive VNS, and it was able to prove something spectacular in the area of VNS as a means of treatment or alternative therapy void of chemicals. The stimulation was discovered to significantly reduce inflammation in patients with rheumatoid arthritis, which worked to inhibit cytokine production, and fostered improved outcomes for these patients.

Rheumatoid arthritis is a major, chronic inflammatory and disabling autoimmune disease that occurs when inflammation damages joints. Rheumatoid arthritis affects about 1.3 million Americans annually, and the treatment costs billions of dollars each year. During the study, the experts involved were able to identify the neural circuitry in charge of regulating inflammation. In one of the circuits, it was discovered that on-going actions transmitted in the vagus nerve was able to stall the production of pro-inflammatory cytokines. What the study finally established was that vagus nerve stimulation has the ability to inhibit the production of cytokine and also weakens the seriousness of acute inflammation in rheumatoid arthritis.

But it's not only in rheumatoid arthritis that vagus nerve stimulation works wonders. In fact, it shows great potential in the treatment of addiction to substance use, for treatment-resistant depression, and for easing physical and emotional pain. Most of these treatment methods that vagus nerve stimulation works with are mostly all the non-invasive methods of VNS. The next chapter is going to look at vagus nerve stimulation as a learned method employed in inhibiting drug addiction in order to stall the risk of relapse.

Chapter Seven

Vagus Nerve Stimulation therapy – a means to Facilitate Extinction Learning

Extinction learning in drug addiction is characterized by learning a new behavior to inhibit the response of a previously learned stimulus, and to prevent the risk of a further relapse into the previous addictive behavior. This is based on information that that points to VNS as a treatment process with the potential to induce cortical plasticity which has a high potential to enhance the extinction of fear memories, and can also work better than drug-based treatments for addiction to substance use. Using VNS in this way, it was discovered that it works in line with those areas of the brain that support the withdrawal and extinction processes of addiction memories. In more clearer terms, this is to say that vagus nerve stimulation therapy has a higher potential of aiding people overcome addiction to drugs by bring to their knowledge that there are other ways to learn behaviors that will replace those associated with the craving for drugs.

The preclinical study was carried out by a group of researchers and Dr. Sven Kroener, who is one of them, has this to say: "We are studying extinction learning and how vagus nerve stimulation can help subjects learn a new behavior that is opposed to an existing, maladaptive behavior like drug taking. When a subject is addicted to a drug, extinction is a method to help them re-learn behaviors – so they are able to take different actions."

When the research team of Dr. Sven Kroener applied vagus nerve stimulation to a group of cocaine addicted laboratory rats used in the research called "extinction learning," they discovered that the stimulation was able to help the animals acquire different behaviors that reduced their cravings for the drug. This was achieved by the changes that were initiated in their brain. This is how it worked. The rats were able to experience specific changes that occurred in the synaptic plasticity between the prefrontal cortex and the amygdala. What the research revealed was that vagus nerve stimulation has the ability to extinguish addictive memories just like it was able to extinguish fearful memories, by rewriting the already written exposure to drugs as the brain has come to know it by introducing new and health rewarding behaviors.

Although it's still a study yet to be fully experimented on humans, the result of the experiment carried out on drug addicted laboratory rats returned with positive outcome. It showed that vagus nerve stimulation has the potency to treat people who are addicted to drugs, by introducing them to new stimulus that will replace the previous one. During the study, the rats, having already been separated into two groups, were kept in a place where they were fed the drug during each session.

Both groups were administered the drug, but only one group were stimulated through new learned behavior.

In both groups, there was a lever and the rats had learned by association how to press it, that upon each pressing the rats received the drug along with light and sound that accompanied the administration. Coupled with the effect of the drug and the heightened ecstasy the music and light gave them, the addictive stimulus was great. But after a while, for one group subsequent sessions did not produce the drug, the light and sound, and due to the associated cues the craving for the drug was enormous in that group. And this was the beginning of vagus nerve stimulation therapy.

They kept pressing the lever for their reward, but nothing happened. In subsequent sessions, it was discovered that, after the initial heightened sense of craving, rats that were undergoing VNS therapy pressed the lever less frequently than those who were still being fed the drug.

What the study recorded was that with time, the number of times they pressed the lever kept reducing per session, until it was only a few times. Then the light and sound was returned but never the drug. They went back to pressing frequently because they remembered the reward they got from the drug. But it wasn't there. What happened was that they got used to the light and sound without the drug. This is how the extinction process works. The rats were able to learn new behaviors through another stimulus, and the addiction to drugs was handled without the help of chemicals. This is exactly what vagus nerve stimulation hopes to achieve with humans when it would be finally used as an extinction process for addictive behavior. To this, Dr. Sven Kroener opined that "The VNS treatment might reinforce abstinence, eventually weaning them off the drug-related behavior and protecting them better from the cravings."

To extinguish fearful memories and drug-seeking memories relies on creating a completely new pathway in the brain, which will be a new stimulus that will have new learned behaviors erode and replace old ones. Hence, the research proved that vagus nerve stimulation has the ability to facilitate the extinction learning process (that's entering a state of complete forgetfulness, just like a slate wiped clean), and it will also inhibit the risk of further relapse. This means that for an addict to overcome their addiction, they have to learn new behaviors that have the magnitude of attraction enough to compete with the addictive behavior.

How Vagus Nerve Stimulation Therapy works

With regard to the magnitude of its role, VNS is a veritable tool in the non-chemical treatment of diseases and health conditions such as epilepsy and depression. And in the case of extinction process during addiction, what the therapy is certain to do is to significantly reduce the craving for the drug, and not to annihilate the symptom of the addiction. Although with a continuous trail, the symptom of addictive behavior will be completely dropped. The complete turnaround from the behavior is as a result of two things: the giant role the nerve plays as the most prominent nerve in the body, and its connection with how the brain works.

Thus stimulating the vagus nerve to treat addiction through electric pulses ensures that those cravings got cut back on as a result of what the vagus nerve can do, and this also works in line with the nerve's influence to eliminate the established connection between taking the drug and the assumed reward it gives. This will completely annihilate the need to take more drugs because there wouldn't be any established reward its consumption promises, and there wouldn't be any experience of reward when it's taken. Dr. Sven Kroener captured this in his words: "That's what you want in addiction treatment. You want to have less craving and less responsiveness to the old cues and the old environment that previously signified drug taking. [Therefore] When a subject is addicted to a drug, extinction is a method to help them relearn behaviors – so they are able to take different actions," and as an addition, the different actions are expected to enable the addict learn new behaviors that will help them reduce or completely forsake drug cravings.

Vagus nerve stimulation therapy is basically a surgical process that's why it's termed an invasive procedure. It works by having a device implanted in the body and connecting it to a wire threaded along the vagus nerve which travels all the way from the neck to the brain, linking the area of the brain that controls mood. The role of the dollar-shaped device is to do the work of an intercessor or better still, a peace maker. It does its job by sending mild electrical impulses to the brain; an impulse that regulates the craving and urge for drug intake.

Chapter Eight

Vagus Nerve Stimulation for Treatment-Resistant Depression

Counting from the most recent years to this point, major scientific discoveries have witnessed changes and findings in neurostimulation treatments for clinical depression, especially for major depressive disorder, and for other disorders such as bipolar disorder. Usually an effective treatment for these mental conditions, the immense benefits of vagus nerve stimulation as an augmentative therapeutic process for treatment-resistant depression patients promises to be felt in the body over a long-term period.

The stimulation of the left cervical vagus as a form of treatment for depression was originally or first employed in the treatment of seizures such as epilepsy. And after it recorded success in this field, it was experimented and the result turned out to be promising for patients with acute treatment-resistant depression. From the earlier experiments it was discovered that treatment-resistant depression patients responded to vagus nerve stimulation therapy just the way they should have responded to antidepressants.

Major depressive disorder is a prevalent mental disease affecting about two out of every ten persons. It is associated with intense feelings of sadness, despair, uselessness, hopelessness, helplessness and non-challant attitude towards life. People suffering major depressive disorder find it difficult to eat, sleep or take active part in social activities, which makes them mostly withdrawn from other people and life in general. Although there are standard antidepressants available as suitable treatments, there are still people who have not been able to respond to the treatment given to them with these antidepressants.

The condition whereby a patient suffering depression is unable to respond to treatment is termed "treatment-resistant depression." And because of this, an effective non-chemical based treatment has been sourced for and that discovered way is vagus nerve stimulation, which was approved sometime in 2005 by the Food and Drugs Administration.

The aim of vagus nerve stimulation as a non-chemical based therapy for MDD is to enhance mood regulation and reduce the acute sadness that comes with depression by stimulating the nerve within the neck that transmits signals in the brain areas involved.

The stimulation works by attaching bipolar electrodes on the left cervical vagus nerve, which is then attached to an implanted stimulator generator through an incision made on the left side of the neck, and then a tiny wire, which is placed under the skin, runs from the device to the vagus nerve in the neck. What the device does is to send out electrical impulses into the nerve, which are then transmitted to the brain. And for some reasons which are beyond medical explanation, but are very much real, the electrical impulses transmitted through the vagus nerve to the brain has been proved to relieve the symptoms of depression, especially for those who are treatment-resistant.

This outcome was reached based on a study carried out sometime on 2005, when a total number of 124 persons who received what the study termed "treatment as usual" (TAU; which could be a combination of antide-pressants, psychotherapy, transcranial magnetic stim-ulation, electroconvulsive therapy, or any other ther-apy) were compared with 205 persons who received treatment as usual alongside vagus nerve stimulation, and over a year period it was proved that there was more improvement on the part of those who combined usual treatment with vagus nerve stimulation when re-garded with those who received only treatment as usual. This goes to show that treating major depressive disorder with usual antidepressants is good, if the treatment proves effective and is able to provide the re-lief it should. But in a case where a patient shows signs of treatment-resistance, a combination of vagus nerve therapy and treatment as usual will be beneficial.

What the Conway Study Revealed

The words of the principal investigator and director of the vagus nerve stimulation – treatment-resistant de-pression study, Dr. Charles R. Conway, a Washington

University professor of psychiatry: "When evaluating patients with treatment-resistant depression, we need to focus more on their overall well-being. A lot of patients are on as many as three, four, or five antidepressant medications and they're just barely getting by. But when you add a vagus nerve stimulator, it really can make a big difference in people's everyday lives," revealed that vagus nerve stimulation is a veritable way of conducting non-chemical based therapies that will yield great results in treatment-resistant depression.

The study which had 328 patients had some of them using only treatment as usual, while the other group had treatment as usual and vagus nerve stimulators also implanted. After a period of time, the group led by Conway evaluated the progress of the participants based on a 14 category scale termed "quality of life factor," which included physical health, family and social relationships, response and reaction to workplace relationship and scenarios, and their well-being as a whole.

What the group discovered was that those who had the vagus nerve stimulator implanted did better than those who did not. They reported a general better feel at life and were more optimistic than those who did not have the stimulator implanted. This finding and progress prompted Conway to say that "On about 10 of the 14 measures, those with vagus nerve stimulators did better. For a person to be considered to have responded to a depression therapy, he or she needs to experience a 50 percent decline in his or her standard depression score. But we noticed, anecdotally, that some patients with stimulators reported they were feeling much better even though their scores were only dropping 34 to 40 percent."

The most important discovery of the Conway led study remains the amazing way the brain controls and reacts to man-made treatment devices through electrical charges. The brain being an electrical organ often requires electrical interaction during its treatment. And being also that depression is a problem of the brain, and even though drugs could be used to treat it, in a case where medications prove abortive, it's best to resort to the things the organ recognizes and understand, which could be in the likes of vagus nerve stimulation. The best part of it comes not only in its electrical interaction with the brain, but also in its potential to functionally cure the neurological condition without zero side effects that comes with medication.

The promise of cure and effective management of symptom which vagus nerve stimulation therapy for treatment-resistant depression avails patients is a life-changing and live-saving progress. It will reduce the level and frequency of suicidal ideation that comes with depression, there will be hope for patient's recovery, and life and living will look promising for them.

Chapter Nine

Vagus Nerve Stimulation: How does it Ease Emotional Pain?

Most emotional pain is caused by untreated or badly treated post-traumatic stress disorder (PTSD). The disorder is the outcome of a badly handled traumatic emotional experience. When you have post-traumatic stress disorder, you are likely to feel pain, fear, uncertainty and anxious when you remember a past experience. Most times the remembrance is intrusive and negative in its core, leaving you with negative thoughts and chronic pain. The most frequently used methods of treatment for the disorder is often a combination of antidepressants, psychotherapy and anti-anxiety medications. Post-traumatic stress disorder has a direct link with pain and mental health.

Because of its unique involvement with pain and the brain, studies and researches were carried out to find out how stimulating the vagus nerve can help ease the pain caused by intrusive negative thoughts and memories. Hence, in a recent study published in February 13, 2019, Imanuel Lerman, an MD, an associate professor at University of California, San Diego School of Medicine; Jacobs School of Engineering and Qualcomm Institute, and a pain management specialist at University of California, San Diego Health and Veterans Affairs, San Diego Healthcare System, and his colleague, Alan

N. Simmons, who is a director of the FMRI Research Laboratory at Veterans Affairs, San Diego Healthcare System, and also an associate professor of psychiatry at University of California, San Diego School of Medicine, made committed efforts to find out how the emotional pain people experience might be improved or influenced by the vagus nerve.

What they did was to test the efficacy of non-invasive vagus nerve stimulation as a means of dampening the sensations of pain by making use of functional magnetic resonance imaging (FMRI) to study what goes on in the brains of thirty healthy participants in a bid to find out what will happen right after a painful heat stimulus was applied to their legs. And also as a means of determining how the sympathetic nervous system responds to pain, the sweat on the skin of the participants were measured before the stimulating heat was applied, and the sweat was equally measured at intervals as the heat increased.

The participants were divided into two equal groups and one group was treated with noninvasive vagus nerve stimulation for two minutes. The treatment was carried out by having electrodes placed on their necks before the heat stimulus was applied ten minutes later, while the other group received what the study termed "mock stimulation." After the electrode was placed and the heat stimulus applied consequently, the team recorded three findings:

Stimulating the vagus nerve via the noninvasive electrode blunted the peak response to heat stimulus in several areas of the brain remarkable for their role in sensory and discriminative pain processing, as well as in most emotional pain points. Another thing the treatment recorded was that the noninvasive stimulation of the vagus nerve delayed the pain response in the emotional pain centers and all the pain regions of the brain. This is to say that the pain related regions of the brain were activated ten seconds later in the participants in the group that were pre-treated with electrodes than those who were sham-treated.

The second finding was in the area of sweating. The sweat measurement revealed that vagus nerve stimulation altered the autonomic responses to painful heat stimulus. And because they didn't experience the pain immediately the heat was applied, they didn't sweat and palpitate with the survival instinct. There was not cortisol or adrenaline to make them sweat profusely. And it was also discovered that instead of sweat more because of the sudden pain, the measure of sweat their bodies produced reduced within a short time when compared with the other participants in the second group, who were sham-treated.

The third finding was that stimulating the vagus nerve equally dampened the sympathetic nervous centers that are responsible for the survival instincts also known as the "fight" or "flight" response. These responses are known to control sweating and accelerated heart rate. But having the electrode stimulate the vagus nerve controlled this.

Although the participants in the stimulated group were grouped under successful experiment, not all of them responded accordingly. Some must have sweated a little more than other, even same as those in the shame treatment. But the major thing is that noninvasive stimulation of the vagus nerve has the tendency to dampen pain and regulate the activities of the pain centers responsible for the feelings and experience of pain. To lay more emphasis on this, Lerman said that "Not everyone is the same. Some people may need more vagus nerve stimulation than other to achieve the same outcomes and the necessary frequencies might change over time."

Invasive and noninvasive Vagus Nerve Stimulation

Vagus nerve stimulation is the use of a device to stimulate the vagus nerve with electrical impulses. The Food and Drug Administration approved invasive stimulation of the vagus nerve for the treatment of ailments like epilepsy and treatment-resistant depression. Now this does not mean that non-resistant patients can't be treated by stimulating the vagus nerve, it means that it functions as an augmentative therapy for "treatment as usual." You have already been told what the vagus nerve is, its role in the body, its location and how helpful its stimulation is. It is equally important that you to learn how to stimulate it.

Usually, to stimulate the vagus nerve a device would have to be implanted in your body, somewhere around your chest region with a wire threaded from the device to connect to the left vagus nerve. And when it's activated, the device will send electrical impulses along your vagus nerve to your brainstem, which in turn will send signals and impulses to certain areas in your brain. The implanted device is connected to your left vagus nerve because the right one functions to carry fibers that supply nerves to your heart.

Then further research revealed that there could be another way to stimulate the vagus nerve without having to involve surgery. Thus the noninvasive stimulation was discovered. The stimulation comprises using a device which is not surgically implanted to stimulate the vagus nerve, and help with the treatment for depression, epilepsy, anxiety and pain. You should note that these ailments mentioned here are not the only ones that could be treated with vagus nerve stimulation therapy; they are just a prototype for discussing the many ailments vagus nerve stimulation can take care of.

The Need for Vagus Nerve Stimulation

Whether as invasive or noninvasive stimulation, there is every need to stimulate the vagus nerve. The reason for this is because more than half of epileptic patients do not respond to anti-seizure drugs; hence, when their vagus nerve is adequately stimulated, the frequency of episodes of seizure will drastically reduce, and it will benefit those who have not been able to record success at control or improvements with medications.

It also proves to be a helpful augmentative or full therapy for treatment-resistant depression patients. There are various treatment approaches available to people with depression, but not all of them are helpful as they should. But when invasive vagus nerve stimulation is used as an approach to treatment, they often record great improvement.

But despite all the helpful reasons why vagus nerve stimulation is a welcome therapy, you should know that it's not for everyone. The Food and Drug Administration has a category of people who could approach vagus nerve stimulation as an alternative, only or augmentative therapy, and they include people who are four years old and above. This means the therapy isn't for infants. It is also approved for people with partial epilepsy, and those who experience seizures that medication couldn't adequately control.

Vagus nerve stimulation is an important discovery in the area of health, and there is every need to include it in treatment-based therapies where medications have proved to be incompetent. But in all that has been discussed about vagus nerve stimulation therapy, there still remains the possibility of side effects. Although it does not involve chemicals and there are almost zero adulterations with it, there is still the possibility that things could go wrong with it. And being that the aim of the book is to discuss vagus nerve stimulation, there is every need to discuss the gains and losses. By doing this, you will be adequately guided in what you do and how you approach it as a treatment-based therapy. The disadvantages would be discussed, and through it you will understand how the disorders come about.

Chapter Ten

The Cons of invasive Vagus Nerve Stimulation Therapy

Vagus nerve stimulation therapy is a worthy process medically approved to help you maintain optimal health status. But in all its goodness, there still remains a chance that it could pose minor and major threat to your wellbeing, depending on the number of things that went wrong during the process. Before you sign up for invasive vagus nerve stimulation, you should consider the following: surgery risks and after surgery side effects.

The surgery risks include complications that might arise during the procedure, and these complications when not adequately handled can lead to long or short-term challenges. The complications can arise from the procedure to implant the device or from stimulating the brain. The risks attached with implanting the device include:

The pain that arose from the point where the incision was made to implant the device. This is typical with all the surgeries, and is not really much of a problem. But it becomes risky if the pain lingers for too long and begins to impair or inhibit day-to-day activities.

The possibility that the laceration might get infected during surgery and implantation. Getting infected might not really pose much threat because ingesting antibiotics can quickly remedy the damage. But if it happens that the infection was not noticed on time, there are chances that it might lead to graver complications.

Since the device is attached somewhere in the chest, there is a possibility that the patient might experience some difficulties when swallowing. The difficulty when not handled can cause other impairments such as a collapse of the vocal cord. Vocal cord paralysis in the case of invasive vagus nerve stimulation is often temporary, but nothing guarantees that it couldn't become permanent if the surgery was not well handled.

These are a few of the surgery risks of invasive vagus nerve stimulation therapy you should look out for. But to deal with these risks and complications that might birth short and long-term side effects, you should fully consider the pros for having the implantation, only then will you decide whether the likely cons are worth the risk. You should consider what your treatment choices are before you decide to have the procedure, and when you have decided you should also acquaint yourself with the possible side effects. You are going to see the possible side effects of invasive vagus nerve stimulation, and then you can decide the way forward.

After-surgery side effects of vagus nerve stimulation

If the surgery goes well and you experience minor complications during surgery, chances are that you might not have many side effects to battle with. But if the procedure is fraught with complications, then there is a higher chance that the side effects might be disastrous. See below some of the after surgery side effects of vagus nerve stimulation:

Because of the nature and manner of the procedure, there is every chance that you might experience voice change. The change in voice might be as a result of the electric impulses on-going in your body, or because of the foreign material lodged somewhere in your core. Whichever one that might be the reason, you should brace yourself that you stand the chance of experiencing voice change after the procedure. This mostly manifests in the likes of hoarseness, and there are other times you might discover that you suddenly began to stutter after the procedure. This might be corrected with little adjustments and with time, and there is also the chance that the fluctuation in voice will remain with you for a lifetime.

There is also a chance that you will develop pain in your throat after the surgery. And there are other times the side effect might be dry and persistent cough followed by headaches and migraine. You could also experience cold shivers, shortness of breath, tingling or prickling of the skin followed by goose bumps, insomnia, and worst case scenario of sleep apnea.

These are a few side effects associated with implanting the device in the case of iVNS. Inasmuch as the side effects concern the procedure for invasive vagus nerve stimulation, they do not apply to everyone who underwent the surgery. The side effects of invasive vagus nerve stimulation behave like the side effects of every other procedure: there are times they are tolerable, and at other times they will remain bothersome until the device is removed. But instead of removing the devices, you can work on adjusting the electrical impulses. Doing this will help with the discomfort, and when it doesn't, you can consider turning it off temporarily or otherwise.

Vagus Nerve Disorder

Just like every other organ in your body, the vagus nerve, though not an organ, can be damaged by some of the activities that destroys organs. Research and studies have shown that chronic alcoholism and diabetes can adversely affect the vagus nerve and even damage it. This because some health challenges lead to the development of foreign or improper bodies in the nerve, and when they stay for too long, they tend to fight their host environment. The time when this damage occurs is not yet known, but symptoms such as bloating, diarrhea, nausea and constipation (gastroparesis) are likely indicators of vagus nerve disorder.

The reason why the disorder has everything to do with the stomach is because the vagus nerve plays an important role in digestion and metabolism. There is also the possibility that the vagus nerve might be destroyed by the presence of a foreign body such as a tumor or physical trauma. These symptoms might lead to conditions like partial or full paralysis of the vocal cords, dry and persistent cough, hoarseness, slowed heart rate, and digestive problems. But the thing is that these manifestations often improve when the tumor is removed or the trauma is handled effectively.

When a disturbance occurs in the vagus nerve, it can cause a whole lot of health challenges such as:

Fainting: Beholding anything that causes your heart to do a summersault is enough to induce fainting. The process of fainting is known as vagal syncope. It is your body responding to the weakness and fatigue caused by stress, trauma and fear. The stress that arises from these things causes an overstimulation of the vagus nerve, which in turn causes a significant drop in your heart rate and blood pressure. If the syncope is extreme or acute, the flow of blood is restricted to your brain, you wouldn't receive adequate blood flow to your legs, and the weakness and numbness will make you lose consciousness. When this happens, it's best you don't try to speed up activities because doing this will make it worse.

Feeling nauseous all the time even in situations that shouldn't permit such feeling. It's understandable that gory sights of death or extreme disgusting situations can trigger nauseous feelings, but having to throw up all the time or feeling that you are going to is not something to overlook. It might signify a problem with the gallbladder, and often time gallbladder problems are linked to the malfunctioning or damage of the vagus nerve. Hence, you might have to check with your doctor.

Unusual weight loss and weight gain are sometimes symptoms of vagus nerve disorder. The weight loss might be as a result of fear of throwing up when you eat, because you are feeling nauseous; hence, you refuse to eat. And at other times the weight gain might be as a result of chronic fatigue, anxiety and depression. You must understand that these symptoms are applicable to anorexia and bulimia nervosa (and sometimes also caused by bingeing); hence, you have to consult your healthcare provider to establish what health problem your weight gain or weight loss indicates. But typically, when an eating disorder is not involved, these manifestations mostly indicate vagus nerve disorder.

Bradycardia and tachycardia are another health challenge caused by vagus nerve disorder. The situation indicates a state where you experience unusual and unwarranted decreased or increased heart rate, respectively. Situations like this can make life unbearable and burdensome. Imagine a scenario where you are unable to stand for a longer period of time because you feel extremely weak, or you experience difficulty walking longer distances because of fatigue. Decreased heart rate causes weakness throughout the joints, whereas increased heart rate feeds the sympathetic nervous system with faux alarm of an imminent danger when there is none. You already know what happens to your health when cortisol is allowed to remain in your system for long.

Irritable bowel syndrome (IBS) is another health hazard that comes with vagus nerve disorder. IBS is a feeling of constant stomach pains and nausea, which renders you uncomfortable and out of shape.

Acute and prolonged depression is also a risk factor of vagus nerve disorder. Because the giant nerve interacts with the brain, when there is a problem with it the brain will also interpret the problem as a threat: hence, the feeling of helplessness and acute sadness that defines depression.

Anxiety is another feeling that comes with vagus nerve disorder. This feeling arises as a result of all the health challenges and disturbances you experience. Some of the disturbances that induce anxiety includes chronic inflammation, fatigue, heartburn, dizziness and the attendant fainting, nausea and the extreme feeling of helplessness, hopelessness and sadness that comes with depression. And because these things are real and manifesting, their presence triggers anxiety.

But to live above anxiety and the problem that caused it (vagus nerve disorder), you can take up activities that promises a lot of reward. There are exercises suitable for stimulating the vagus nerve. Most of them have been mentioned all over the book, but for purpose of clarity they would be listed again. The reason is for you to have a list of exercises that will help you keep your vagus nerve in good health and also maintain a general body optimal balance. Find below to see a list of health and easy-to-do exercises that will stimulate your vagus nerve and help it heal itself of any disorder:

- Deep and slow belly breathing. Instead of breathing fourteen to fifteen times in a minute, you can breathe six to seven times per minute.

- Chanting.

- Cold water bath or face immersion after physical exercise.

- Having your mouth filled with saliva and submerging your tongue in it. Doing this triggers a vagal response.

- Gargling loudly with water in your mouth.

- Singing and laughing loudly.

- Massaging the space between your two ears.

There are a lot more exercises you can do to ensure you stimulate your vagus nerve for a healthy body.

Chapter Ten

Polyvagal Theory

Polyvagal theory clarifies three distinct parts of our nervous system and their reactions to distressing circumstances. When we comprehend those three parts, we can understand why and how we respond to high measures of pressure.

If you think that polyvagal theory sounds as boring as staring at a fly, try to perch repeatedly on a bench, just stay with me. It gets better. It's an interesting clarification of how our body handles emotional pressure, and how we can utilize various therapies to change the impact of trauma.

The Importance of Polyvagal Theory

For therapists, and people who enjoy the field of psychology as well, understanding polyvagal theory can help with:

- Comprehending trauma and PTSD

- Understanding how attack and withdrawal operates in relationships

- Seeing how outrageous stress prompts shutting down or dissociation.

- Seeing how to read non-verbal communication

We like to think about our feelings as ethereal, complex, and hard to classify and distinguish.

In all actuality, feelings are reactions to a stimulus (interior or outside). Frequently they occur out of our mindfulness, particularly in the event that we are withdrawn or incongruent, with our inward emotional life.

Our base desire to remain alive is more important to our body than even our capacity to consider remaining alive. That is the place polyvagal theory comes in to play.

The nervous system is continually running out of sight, controlling our body capacities so we can consider different things—like what sort of frozen yogurt we'd prefer to request, or how to get that A in school. The whole nervous system works together with the brain and can assume control over our emotional experience, regardless of whether we need it to or not.

Below is a short story about a deer to further explain.

Creatures are an incredible case of how we handle pressure, since they respond basely, without mindfulness. They behave just how we would behave if we weren't so all around restrained.

If you have ever viewed a National Geographic Africa special, you've seen a lioness pursue a deer. A herd of deer is touching, and all of a sudden, one turns upward, hyper mindful of what's going on around it. The entire herd notices and focuses.

After a minute, the lioness begins her pursuit. The deer she's singled out runs as quickly as possible until it is gotten (a product of the sympathetic nervous system). At the point when it is gotten, it quickly goes limp (a product of the parasympathetic sensory system).

The lioness hauls the deer back to her offspring, where they start to play with it before they go in for the kill. On the off chance that the lioness gets occupied, and the deer sees a snapshot of chance, it's up and dashing off once more, appearing as though it abruptly returned to life (once more a product of the sympathetic nervous system).

At the point when the deer was gotten, with teeth around his neck, its shutdown reaction kicked in—it became still. At the point when it saw the chance to run, its fight or flight kicked in, and it ran.

Polyvagal hypothesis covers those three states—association, fight or flight, or shutdown.

Association state

During non-stressful circumstances, if we are genuinely still, our bodies remain in a social commitment state, or a glad, ordinary, non-go nuts state. This state can be referred to as association. What is implied by "association" is that we are equipped for an "associated" collaboration with another person. We are strolling close, unafraid, making the most of our day, eating with loved ones, and our body and feelings feel typical.

It's additionally called ventral vagal reaction since that is the part of the mind that is enacted during association mode. It resembles a green light for typical life.

This looks and feels like the following:

- Our immune system is sound.

- We feel ordinary joy, transparency, harmony, and interest in existence.

- We are resting soundly and eating normally.

- Our face is expressive.

- We genuinely identify with others.

- We all the more effectively comprehend and tune in to other people.

- Our body feels quiet and grounded.

Stop, run, fight, or swell upstate

The sympathetic nervous system is our quick response to stress that influences almost every organ in the body.

The sympathetic nervous system causes that flight and fight state we have all known about. It gives us those signs with the goal that it can keep us alive.

This feels like the following:

- We sense risk and stop to examine the surroundings for genuine threats.

- We release cortisol, epinephrine, and norepinephrine to enable us to achieve what we have to—escape or battle our foe.

- Our pulse spikes, we sweat, and we feel more activated.

- We feel restless, apprehensive, or irate.

- There might be flashes of outward appearances of dread and outrage, with the foundation of to a greater extent a still face. In the event that positive feelings are available, they typically look constrained.

- Our absorption backs off as blood hurries to the muscles.

- Our veins contract to the digestion tracts and enlarge to the muscles expected to run or battle.

- Our hands might be sticky.

- We might need to flee, or punch somebody, or respond physically somehow or another, or simply buff-up and look threatening.

- Every one of our faculties focuses.

- Our signals may show guarding of our imperative organs, clench hands gripped or puffing ourselves up to look greater or more grounded.

- Our stomach might be horrendously tied.

- In battle or flight, at some level, we accept we can at present endure whatever risk we believe would save us.

Shutdown state

What's intriguing about this piece of the parasympathetic nervous system? It is its capacity to keep us still as a versatile component to assist us with getting by to either battle or flight once more.

At the point when our sympathetic nervous system has kicked into overdrive, regardless of if we can't escape and feel approaching demise, the dorsal vagal parasympathetic nervous system takes control.

It causes stilling or shutdown, as a part of self-safeguarding. (Consider somebody who falls under extraordinary stress.)

This looks and feels like the following:

- Inwardly, it feels like separation, deadness, mixed-up feelings, misery, disgrace, a feeling of being caught, out of body, detached from the world

- Our eyes may appear fixed and spread apart

- The dorsal engine core through the unmyelin- ated vagus nerve diminishes our pulse, circula- tory pressure, outward appearances, sexual and immune reaction systems

- We might be activated to feel nauseated, vomit, poop, and immediately pee

- We may feel low or no pain.

- Our lungs (bronchi) choke, and we inhale slower.

- We may experience issues getting words out or feel narrowing around our throat.

- Our mind has diminished digestion, and this causes lost body mindfulness, limp appendages, diminished capacity to think plainly, and dimin- ished capacity to set down memory recollec- tions.

- Our body stance may fall or twist up in a ball.

In shutdown mode, at some level, our sensory system accepts we are in a perilous circumstance, and it at- tempts to keep us alive through keeping our body still.

A few people who have had both connection trauma and the resulting trauma can have interminable sui- cidal, and dissociation episodes that range from days to months. Research shows that long haul treatments in- clude:

- Mentalization-based therapy

- Dialectical behavioral therapy

- Transference focused therapy

The Effects of Trauma on Nervous System and Its Relationship with Polyvagal Theory.

As people, we behave in a similar way as that deer when we see emotional or physical risk. We shift back and forth between serene behavior (parasympathetic - association mode), fight or flight (sympathetic - fight and flight mode), or shutdown (parasympathetic-shut down mode).

Our reaction is all in our impression of the occasion. Possibly somebody was simply playing a game when they hopped out to terrify us. However, we blacked out. Whatever the explanation, regardless of whether the episode was purposeful or not, our body moved into shutdown mode, we registered it as a trauma; our body moved into shutdown mode.

Or then again, perhaps the trauma occasion was truly, perilous, and our nervous system reacted suitably to the upgrades.

Regardless of what the reason was, our mind accepted what was going on was perilous enough that it made our body go into flight, fight, or shutdown mode.

In the event that somebody has experienced such a horrible occurrence, that their body tips into shutdown reaction, any occasion that helps the individual to remember that perilous event can trigger them into dissociation or shut down once more.

Individuals can even live in a condition of dissociation or shut down for a considerable length of time or months one after another.

War veterans regularly experience this during noisy, abrupt clamors, for example, firecrackers or tempests. A lady who was assaulted may rapidly switch into the hypervigilant or dissociated reaction in the event that she feels somebody is following her.

The issue happens when we haven't handled the first trauma so that the first trauma is settled.

That is the thing that PTSD (Post Traumatic Stress Disorder) is—our body's eruption to a little reaction, and being either stuck in fight or flight mode or shut down mode.

Individuals who experience trauma and the shutdown reaction, as a rule, feel disgrace around their powerlessness to act, when their body didn't move. They frequently wish they would have fought more during those minutes.

A war veteran may feel they bombed their mates who passed on around them while they stood, frozen in dread. A victim of rape may feel the individual in question didn't fend off their attacker since they froze. An abuse victim may feel they quit attempting to get away from their abuser, and that they are frail or weak.

A lot of "stress" preparing, which trains individuals to keep on staying in fight and flight mode, intends to keep individuals out of dissociation during permanent or passing circumstances. Tragically, these practices aren't normal past high-performance sports teams or special forces. The perfect measure of worry, with great recuperation, can lead our nervous systems into more elevated levels of adjustment.

Leaving shutdown mode

Stepping away from shutdown mode using the Polyvagal theory is important. So how would we move away from shutdown mode?

Something contrary to the dorsal vagal system is the social commitment system.

Along these lines, to put it plainly, what fixes shutdown mode is bringing somebody into solid social commitment, or legitimate connection.

Getting down into the stray pieces of how this functions in our body can assist us with understanding why we feel the way we do physically when your body is in fight, flight, or shut down mode.

At the point when we comprehend why our body responds in the manner in which it does, similar to a series of intimations and some essential science about the mind, we can see how to switch states. We can start to move out of the fight or flight state, out of the shutdown mode, and over into the social commitment state.

Realizing how to explore the polyvagal states is very necessary.

It can likewise be useful if you have quite recently recognized yourself in a portion of these indications. For example, "When I'm with my folks, even as a grown-up and they start fighting, I feel bleary-eyed and disengaged."

On the off chance that you've seen a portion of these things in yourself, ideally through treatment, and in any event, seeing how this works, you can haul yourself out of a disengaged state.

Studies show that a few parts of the mind shut down during the review of awful mishaps, including the verbal focuses and the thinking focuses of the cerebrum.

This is the reason it's imperative to lead treatment on leaving shutdown mode, in a sheltered, sound way, in a protected, solid condition. This is the reason positive connection is basic. Else, you risk re-traumatizing the person struggling with the trauma.

In this segment of the chapter, I am writing this to show how to enable a victim of trauma or anxiety to come out of shutdown mode.

In any case, these tips still apply to the individuals who are simply seeing how shutdown mode functions. Furthermore, it can even enable individuals who feel shut down to start to realize how to attempt to achieve a sound social commitment mode once more.

- Have a trust-based relationship. Due to the possibility to re-traumatize, don't address strongly horrible accidents—particularly ones where you think shutdown mode kicked in until the remedial relationship feels profoundly associated.

- It's significant as the therapist to enable the victim to express things they couldn't express to others—disgraceful emotions, outrage, sexual reaction, anything that feels alarming to tell other people.

- Locate your own quiet focus. On the off chance that you can sympathize with their pain, remain at the time with them, and assist them with feeling associated during their shutdown, you are tossing them a lifesaver. You're helping them leave shutdown, into social commitment.

- It's critical to battle against the desire to dissociate, regardless of how frightful the topic is. As a therapist or person helping out a victim, you could dissociate as a result of the mirror neuron reaction—to reflect the person's mental state, and in light of the fact that when hearing horrendous trauma, it's anything but difficult to envision it transpiring.

The human experience is ground-breaking to such an extent that when we reconnect the trauma, with another person to help us, it revises that occasion in our mind, including the sentiment of being upheld inside the trauma memory. We make new neural pathways around the injury, and we can change our body's reaction to it.

- Allow the person in need of help lead. Try not to go on a witch chase. On the off chance that the patient brings it up, incline toward the subject. In any case, it is destructive to provoke the patient into something that isn't there by posing driving inquiries and attempting to get them to admit. Try not to give your very own experience a chance to lead you to envision they have additionally experienced something.

- Help them understand that their reaction is normal. The whole polyvagal theory should make us state "thank you!" to our bodies. Regardless of the fact that the systems in our bodies are over-active now and again—unjustifiable frenzy or uneasiness—, it is also true that our body is looking out for us, attempting to keep us alive.

Our body responding in that manner is a similar thing as the deer either fleeing or going limp. What's more, deer have no clue what feelings are in any case.

Since the patient comprehends that their emotional reaction was versatile, base, and suitable, we can dispose of the disgrace that their non-response caused.

- Assist them with finding their outrage. Outrage is an unimaginably versatile feeling, and it's one we don't enable ourselves to have. We think outrage is terrible. However, outrage gives us power over where our sound limits were reached.

Outrage gives us vitality to defeat the hindrance. We can help the person who has been through trauma see they had the passionate vitality to survive, yet the vitality couldn't be shown at the time they needed it.

If, in a session, we can get someone who has experienced trauma to recognize their displeasure, they will see that they were not totally lethargic to the horrendous mishap. If we can enable them to feel even the most diminutive development of a microexpression of outrage all over—the slight downturn of the internal eyebrows—we can show them their body didn't thoroughly sell them out at that time.

We can reconnect their body and their sentiments to their feelings. This builds up a condition of coinciding—where their inside sentiments coordinate their external shows of those emotions.

Furthermore, as a dissociative memory is investigated, discovering outrage and lessening disgrace in associatoon with the memory, causes the memory to-on a very basic level-change. Outrage brings them out of separation, regardless of whether it is outrage at you, the therapist, or someone else.

- Present body development. Since shutdown makes us freeze, reactivating body developments while discussing the injury is an incredible method to reconnect the body and mind, to bring them out of shutdown.

For instance, there was a case of an individual who was in an accident. At the point when the emergent response people appeared, they tied him to a gurney to stack him into the back of a rescue vehicle. More than the genuine mishap, being caught on that gurney was horrendous for him. For the whole ride to the emergency clinic, he was startled that he had hurt his neck, and the entirety of the nervousness that encompasses neck damage made him be frozen in dread.

Indeed, even in discussing the injury in the treatment session, his body was hardened, solidified, and he was dissociating.

The therapist asked him, "How might you have needed to move during that minute?" He said he would have needed his arms to have the option to move. The therapist asked him to gradually, carefully, move his arms in the manner in which he would have needed to.

It's essential to do the development carefully and gradually, concentrating on the vibe of the development. That patient felt an immense arrival of vitality. In the accompanying sessions, he had the option to tell the memory as a story, rather than dissociating.

Having the patient move—slow punching, kicking, bending, running gradually—flips the individual from shutdown into the fight or flight mode, with the objective being to move into association, or social commitment, mode.

Body development workouts, related to conversing with a specialist, can, on a very basic level, change the memory.

- Rehearsing confidence. The emotional shutdown can happen inside connections where one individual feels they can't speak with the other individual well.

One specialist, John Gottman, depicts this training as stonewalling. Rehearsing empathy can help the patient feel more responsible for their emotional state, and have a sense of security to move into sound relationship designs.

- Breathwork, care, and yoga all have a job in getting increasingly associated with your present time, place and body.

- Become a master at martial art and practice quality training. This resets the stress system after some time. Further accomplishing something hard, on a progressing premise, takes into account building inward quality, which can keep you in fight and flight longer before going into shut down.

Conclusion

Are you still in uncertain of what the vagus nerve can do or what it represents in the anatomy of your body? Well, that should be anymore if you actually read this book. You have seen how the giant nerve in the body makes you function effectively and how a problem with it affects you in the ways you never imagined possible. Now you have understood how it can help you with health conditions that prove resistant to medications and how it makes life worth living, regardless of the troubles associated with addiction, depression, epilepsy, anxiety, and pain.

The vagus nerve is an all time important nerve in the body, and stimulating makes it all the more important.